Virtual Reality, Real Emergency

In an effort to investigate the revolutionary potential of augmented reality (AR) and virtual reality (VR) technologies in the field of mechanical and medical emergency management, *Virtual Reality, Real Emergency* was written. This book seeks to educate readers on how AR and VR may transform response to emergencies, boost training, and facilitate better decision-making under pressure. It aims to equip professionals and hobbyists alike to use these immersive technologies for saving lives and minimizing calamities by analyzing real-world applications, cutting-edge breakthroughs, and practical insights.

The ground-breaking book *Virtual Reality, Real Emergency: Integrating AR/VR in Computing and Medical Crisis Management* has two goals: to teach and to give readers agency in times of crisis. Our goal is to educate both industry experts and casual observers on the revolutionary possibilities of AR and VR in the high-stakes arenas of mechanical and medical emergency response. The gap between theory and practice is something we want to close by providing real-world insights, practical counsel, and examples of achievement. Our goal is to educate the public on the potential life-saving benefits of AR and VR technology, demystify these tools for the general reader, and provide concrete measures for incorporating them into existing emergency response procedures.

This book not only celebrates the technological advances that have been accomplished but also calls for more cooperation to ensure that these innovations are implemented in a way that puts people's lives first during emergencies.

Virtual Reality, Real Emergency

Integrating AR/VR in Computing and Medical Crisis Management

Edited by
Arvind Dhaka
Farid Nait-Abdesselam
Amita Nandal
Dijana Capeska Bogatinoska
Pramod Singh Rathore
Arpit Kumar Sharma
Dmytro Zubov

CRC Press
Taylor & Francis Group
Boca Raton London New York

CRC Press is an imprint of the
Taylor & Francis Group, an **informa** business

Designed cover image: Shutterstock Images

First edition published 2026
by CRC Press
2385 NW Executive Center Drive, Suite 320, Boca Raton FL 33431

and by CRC Press
4 Park Square, Milton Park, Abingdon, Oxon, OX14 4RN

CRC Press is an imprint of Taylor & Francis Group, LLC

ISBN: 978-1-032-93208-8 (hbk)
ISBN: 978-1-032-93209-5 (pbk)
ISBN: 978-1-003-56490-4 (ebk)

DOI: 10.1201/9781003564904

Typeset in Minion
by SPi Technologies India Pvt Ltd (Straive)

Contents

Editors

Arvind Dhaka (PhD) received his PhD in computer science and engineering from NIT Hamirpur, India, in 2018. Currently he is Associate Professor in the Department of Computer and Communication Engineering at Manipal University Jaipur. He has more than 40 research papers, out of which 30 are in top-rated SCI indexed journals. He completed one research project funded by DST New Delhi in 2023.

Farid Nait-Abdesselam (PhD) is Professor in the Department of Computer Science, Paris Cité University, Paris, France. His research interests include security and privacy, networking, Internet of Things, and healthcare systems. He has authored/co-authored over 150 research papers in these areas. He received his PhD degree from University of Versailles, France.

Amita Nandal (PhD) received her PhD in electronics and communication engineering from SRM University, Chennai, in 2014. Currently she is Professor in the Department of IoT and Intelligent Systems, Manipal University Jaipur. She has more than 50 research papers, out of which 30 are in top-rated SCI indexed journals. She completed one research project funded by DST New Delhi in 2023.

Dijana Capeska Bogatinoska (PhD) received her PhD in applied computer science from St. Clement of Ohrid University of Bitola, Faculty of Information and Communication Technologies, Bitola, Republic of Macedonia, in 2023. Since 2022, she is working as Associate Professor in the University of Information Science and Technology "St. Paul the Apostle" (UIST) – Ohrid, Republic of Macedonia.

Pramod Singh Rathore (PhD) received his PhD in computer science and engineering from UEM, Jaipur, India, in 2023. Currently he is working in the Department of Computer and Communication Engineering at

Manipal University Jaipur, Jaipur, India. With over 13 years of academic teaching experience, he has published more than 85 papers in reputable, peer-reviewed national and international journals, books, and conferences. He is a senior member of IEEE, member of ACM, and member of International Association of Engineers (IAENG).

Arpit Kumar Sharma (PhD) received his PhD in computer and communication engineering from Manipal University Jaipur, India, in 2023. Since 2022, he is working as Assistant Professor in the Department of Computer and Communication Engineering at Manipal University Jaipur. His research interests include medical image processing and machine learning and deep learning in image processing.

Dmytro Zubov (PhD) is Associate Professor of computer science based at the University of Central Asia's Naryn campus. His PhD was validated in China and North Macedonia. His certificates and awards include Microsoft Server Virtualization Professional with Windows Server Hyper-V and System Center, and Microsoft Azure Research Award in 2014 and 2016. He also holds memberships at Microsoft, IBM, and IEEE. In his educational activities, Dr. Zubov focuses on mobile apps based on the Java Android and offline HTML5+JavaScript+CSS technologies, Internet of Things/Everything (IoT/E), and responsive Bootstrap websites. Dr. Zubov is a leader of the Smart City Mesh Network of eHealth Intelligent Agents for Visually Impaired and Blind People international project. His main research goals are aimed at creating intelligent agents in IoT/E systems such as smart energy, smart industry, smart buildings, and inclusive smart assistive infrastructure for the visually impaired and blind people (Java Android apps, Raspberry Pi, and Arduino/Genuino hardware with different sensors/actuators, SIFT image processing, MQTT IoT protocol, and WiFi/Ethernet technologies). He has experience in developing HPC applications in the public (Windows Azure) and private (Windows Server) computing clouds.

Contributors

Venkata Krishna Azith Teja Ganti
Microsoft Corporation
Charlotte, NC, USA

Thulasi Bikku
Department of Computer Science and Engineering
Amrita School of Computing
Amaravati, India

M. Clement Joe Anand
Department of Mathematics
Mount Carmel College (Autonomous)
Bengaluru, India

Govinda Rajulu G
Department of Computer Science and Engineering
Vel Tech Rangarajan Dr. Sagunthala R&D Institute of Science and Technology
Chennai, India

Sk Hasane Ahammad
KL University, Green Fields
Guntur, India

Rajiv U Kalebar
School of Business and Management
Christ University
Bengaluru, India

Harinadh Karimikonda
School of Management Studies
Sreenidhi Institute of Science and Technology
Hyderabad, India

Kavitha G L
Department of Information Science and Engineering
Atria Institute of Technology
Bengaluru, India

Lakshminarayana Reddy Kothapalli Sondinti
US Bank
Dallas, TX, USA

Kalyani S Kumar
Department of Computer Science & Engineering
BNM Institute of Technology
Bangalore, India

K. Madhavi
Department of Commerce
Maharani Women's Arts, Commerce and Management
Kudumula, India

Kiran Kumar Maguluri
Cigna
Plano, TX, USA

Hariballav Mahapatra
Department of Diabetology
Sevayan Diabetes Centre, Shree Hospitals
Bhubaneswar, India

Malini R
Department of Information Science and Engineering
Atria Institute of Technology
Bengaluru, India

Gowtham Mandala
Purdue University
West Lafayette, IN, USA

Vishwanadham Mandala
Cummins Inc.
Greenwood, IN, USA

V.S.N. Murthy
Department of Information Technology
Shri Vishnu Engineering College for Women
Bhimavaram, India

Anitha Nallasivam
FMS, CMS Business School
JAIN (Deemed-to-be University)
Bengaluru, India

Chandrashekar Pandugula
Lowes Inc
Mooresville, NC, USA

Pramoda Patro
School of Computer Science and Artificial Intelligence
SR University
Warangal, India

Guna Sekhar Sajja
Department of Information Technology
University of the Cumberlands
Williamsburg, KY, USA

Santosh Reddy P
Department of Computer Science & Engineering
BNM Institute of Technology
Bangalore, India

Aaluri Seenu
Department of CSE
SVECW
Bhimavaram, India

C Selvaraj
Jain Online, Management Studies
JAIN (Deemed-to-be University)
Bengaluru, India

R. Senthamil Selvan
Department of ECE
Annamacharya Institute of Technology and Sciences
Tirupati, India

Charanjeet Singh
Department of Electronics and Communication
Deenbandhu Chhotu Ram University of Science and Technology
Murthal, India

Kiran Sree Pokkuluri
Department of Computer Science and Engineering
Shri Vishnu Engineering College for Women
Bhimavaram, India

Tulasi Naga Subhash Polineni
Exelon
Baltimore, MD, USA

P.R. Sudha Rani
Department of CSE
SVECW
Bhimavaram, India

Supriya Sudhir
Department of Computer Science & Engineering
BNM Institute of Technology
Bangalore, India

K. Suresh Kumar
Department of MBA
Panimalar Engineering College
Chennai, India

Swetha N
Department of Management
Alliance Ascent College, Alliance University
Bengaluru, India

Breeze Tripathi
Department of Business and Commerce
PSS Central Institute of Vocational Education
Bhopal, India

Ravi Kumar Vankayalapati
Equinix
Dallas, TX, USA

Majjari Venkata Kesava Kumar
Department of EEE
JNTUA
Anantapur, India

Zakera Yasmeen
Microsoft Corporation
Charlotte, NC, USA

CHAPTER 1

The Effect of Virtual Reality Instructors on the Development of Surgical Competence

Thulasi Bikku, K. Suresh Kumar, M. Clement Joe Anand, and Kiran Sree Pokkuluri

1.1 INTRODUCTION

Investing time, money, and specialized supervision into training surgeons is no small feat [1]. Surgical illness burdens are significant in many low- and middle- income countries, yet postgraduate surgical training opportunities are few [2–4]. Surgical training materials may be shared with large, geographically distributed audiences via the use of inexpensive and scalable virtual reality (VR) technology [5]. These include:

- Faculty of specialist surgeons teaching surgical techniques using cadaveric specimens.
- Participants engaged in in-person, practical instruction.
- Content captured with 360-degree video and several stationary camera perspectives.
- Live-streamed content is to distant representatives in a 360-degree perspective [6], with overlays from fixed cameras to provide various views.

DOI: 10.1201/9781003564904-1

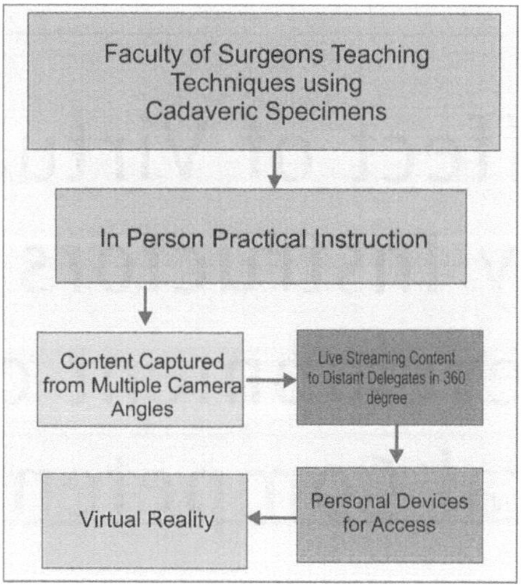

FIGURE 1.1 Virtual reality technology materials.

- Virtual reality headsets with high specifications [7], smartphones with low-cost VR headsets, or smartphones alone are all examples of personal devices that can access VR-content laptops only (360-degree video) [8] (Figure 1.1).

VRiMS first offered five courses designed to meet the requirements of surgical trainees and subsequently modified those courses to meet the demands of surgical training in low- and middle-income countries [9–11]. By utilizing a mixed-method assessment, we provide the results of the first Global VRiMS course [12], which was jointly organized by academic and clinical groups.

1.2 METHODOLOGY

1.2.1 Initial Investigation

A suggested one-day preliminary inquiry included "Bellwether" measures that might save lives. Faculty members imparted knowledge both in-person and online [13]. Nearly thirty-six low- and middle-income countries (LMICs) and seventeen high-income countries (HICs) sent representatives to the free, worldwide live stream. Users were actively involved (with a mean engagement time of over 140 minutes per delegate) [14], however feedback after the course was seldom used.

1.2.2 Creation of Content

Surgical, obstetric, and trauma-related procedures from the World Health Organization's "Essential Surgery Package" served as the basis for the development of the individualized course material via GASOC's (the Global Anaesthesia, Surgery and Obstetrics Collaborative) vast surgical network, which the researchers were able to modify via discussions with rural/remote general practitioners, trainees, and expert surgeons [15–17]. Acquiring 360-degree video while positioned at the operation table allowed for the creation of VR material. Also, regular cameras placed at various positions allowed for simultaneous recording, which allowed for the overlay of many viewpoints [18].

As a result, the live stream showed the whole operating room as a 360-degree panorama, with several typical secure interpretations superimposed as quadrilateral figures in an edging sight [19], as if they were displayed around the table (Figure 1.2).

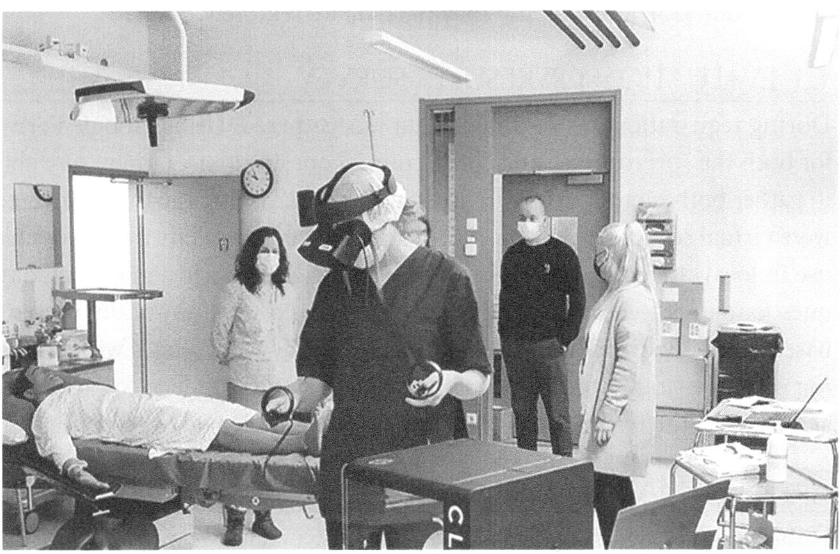

FIGURE 1.2 Operating room as a 360-degree panorama.

1.2.3 Recruiting Delegates

All delegates were required to pre-register, and there were no fees for the courses. Promotions reached students and medical professionals via word-of-mouth, national television, online platforms, and based on interest email lists [20–22]. Information was shared. Three-course delegations were recruited:

- Saving Faces provided an in-person, practical cadaveric training, with scholarships available to assist with expenses, including accommodation [23]. The criteria required to assess eligibility included involvement in medical practice in a low- or middle-income nation, a personal statement, curriculum vitae, surgical logbook, specialized reference letter, and a valid passport [24]. To maximize effect, emphasis was placed on candidates serving extensive, distant, or rural populations, as well as those educating other healthcare professionals.
- Daily in-person virtual training for up to 30 people, smartphone, charger, and headphones; inexpensive wooden VR headsets were provided.
- Virtual training with remote access. Anyone in the world with an internet connection, a 360-degree virtual reality headset, a smartphone [25], and a laptop may participate remotely.

1.3 EVALUATION OF RESULTS SURVEY

During registration, demographic data was gathered. Using Google Forms for both the "pre-course" and "post-course" questionnaires, they were able to gather both quantitative and qualitative data. Among the topics covered were virtual reality's effects on course attendance, accessibility, and possible use in local clinical practice. At the beginning and conclusion of each day, questionnaires were handed out to delegates who were physically present, based on the findings from the pilots that indicated challenges with engaging with post-course feedback. Owing to their significant face-to-face interactions with the research team, this group was anticipated to respond later.

1.4 INFORMAL INTERVIEWS

Fourteen comprehensive semi-structured interviews were used to gather qualitative data. On the last day of the course, all delegates who were physically present were questioned face to face; meanwhile, delegates who were remotely present were interviewed digitally after the course had ended (April–July 2022). Participants in the interviews were given information sheets outlining the goals and parameters of the study, and they were also asked to sign a permission document. Data were analyzed thematically using NVivo after following topic guidance and recording and transcribing interviews word for word. The research was iterative; theoretical considerations and inductive coding led to the development of themes. The dissection lab in the anatomy lab has a Public Display Licence and an HTA Anatomy Licence, which are issued by the Human Tissue Authority (HTA) and are according to The Human Tissue Act 2004.

1.5 RESULTS

Every number is rounded to the nearest tenth of a percent, and all means are given.

1.5.1 Overview of Training Programme

According to the World Health Organization and suggestions from physicians and surgeons, the course content is shown in Table 1.1. After a quick ten-minute talk covering most of the material, delegates worked with real-life examples and cadavers. In cases when the use of real cadavers is neither feasible nor ethical, such as in the case of an obstetric emergency affecting the uterus of a pregnant woman, the Limbs and Things manikins are used as an alternative. Every detail on the program is available online.

TABLE 1.1 Course Content

Title	Delivery Methods	Time Allocated
Essential surgical care access	L	42 Mins.
Trauma epidemiology and management	L	42 Mins.
Save and stabilize: airway	L, C, M	1 Hr. 30 Mins.
Stabilization: breathing, circulation, and vascular access	L, C	3 Hrs. 30 Mins.
Management of wounds and burns	L, C	2 Hrs.
Abdominal trauma management	L, C	2 Hrs.
Emergency and essential abdominal surgery	L, C	3 Hrs. 30 Mins.
The fracture management principles	L, C	2 Hrs.
Limb trauma management	L, C	2 Hrs.
Head trauma management	L, C	3 Hrs. 30 Mins.
Pregnancy complications management	L, C, M	2 Hrs.
Obstetrics/gynaecology emergencies and postpartum haemorrhage	L, C	3 Hrs.

Note: Time and delivery methods discussed throughout the training.
C–Cadaveric procedural demonstrations, L–lecture, and M–manikin demonstrations.

1.5.2 Access Method

Aside from their allotted fifteen minutes for virtual reality, in-person delegates opted for "hands-on" instruction throughout every experiential session. Delegates favoured using inexpensive cardboard headsets in conjunction with their cell phones, spaced out with brief intervals of utilizing the device/computer alone. Due to their immense popularity, the two Oculus headsets were used continuously during the whole course day. One drawback that was noted was the need to periodically charge them. The situation was different with cell phones, however, since they could still be charged while in use.

1.5.3 Demographics of Delegates

Virtual reality was used by delegates with little to no expertise, with just a small number having played games or engaged in other unnamed VR-related activities. There was a disparity between the number of attendees registered on the digital platform and the number of feedback forms completed by distant delegates. This is consistent with the observation that some group members submitted feedback forms from different devices. The post-course feedback did not specifically address this use type as it was not expected. However, the numbers show that most people logged in using only one device. People from many different countries made up the remote group's geographically dispersed workforce.

1.5.4 Information Gathered from Surveys

High participation was reported in the survey for all three-course delegate types: remote or virtual training, in-person hands-on training, and in-person training with VR live-streaming. Even months after the course, those who had hands-on training in person still felt its influence on their clinical practice. Several delegates claimed to apply what they learned daily, and every single delegate did so at least once a month. The majority of delegates said that each delivery mode had a favourable influence on their clinical practice. This was especially true for practical sessions, lectures, and virtual reality learning.

Regarding implementation, delegates from all methodologies saw an uptick in the quality of their patient evaluations and surgical operations. Moreover, without exception, every single participant said they had taught others, and many of them said they do it often. People who watched the live stream shared their thoughts on how easy it was to access the virtual

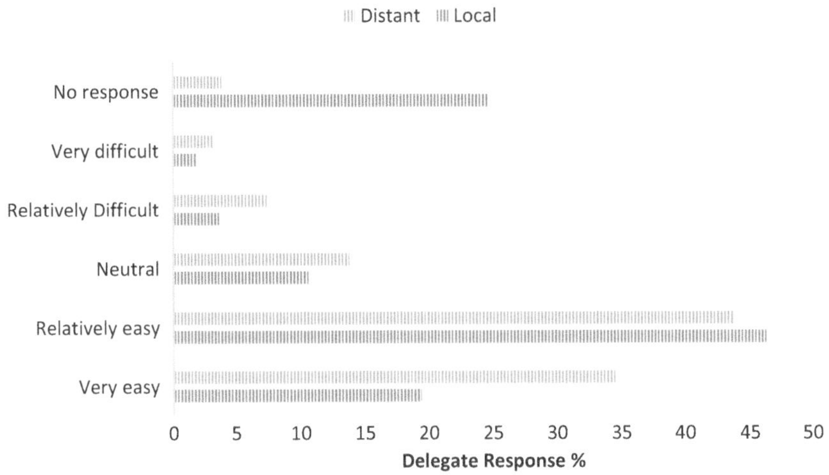

FIGURE 1.3 VR ease of use post-course survey replies from live stream delegates.

reality information, how it increased attendance, and how it might be used for local surgical education and practice. The most significant obstacle to access, as revealed in the survey's free-form parts, was an inadequate internet connection.

Figures 1.3 and 1.4 show the replies from delegates who were either local or distant viewers of the live stream. The majority of participants said that accessing VR information was straightforward or somewhat easy;

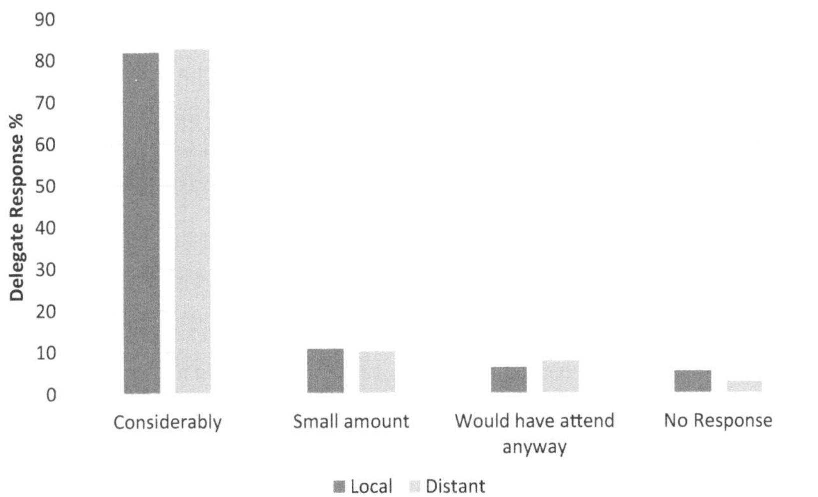

FIGURE 1.4 Post-course survey results from delegates who attended the course via live stream about VR's appeal.

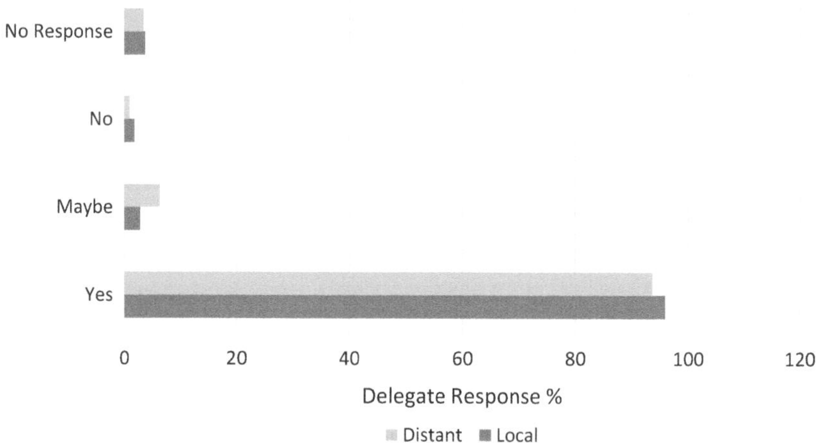

FIGURE 1.5 Live stream delegates' post-course survey replies on VR's usefulness.

that the virtual reality component of the sequence encouraged them to attend; and that they believe virtual reality may be useful in local surgical education, training, and practice (Figure 1.5).

1.5.5 Semi-Formal Interviews

Based on the participant interviews, three main themes emerged: first, the study's background regarding the problem of medical training and ability development; second, how VR could assist with this via its 360-degree visualization and integrated knowing-as-seeing mechanism; and third, the persistent problems regarding the accessibility and acceptability of VR in surgical education. Notably, interviews were conducted in English, and although participants were expected to be proficient in the language, most did not speak it as their first language.

1.5.6 Training for Healthcare Professionals

Many interviewees said they do surgical operations using just what they learned in their bachelor's degree programs since there are so few options for postgraduate training in their own countries. Medical institutions may not always back their graduates' efforts to further their careers once they graduate. When people are responsible for paying for their education, they may feel less incentive to keep their skills current and may even be less motivated to do so. A participant said that they sometimes use what they learned in undergrad to do little surgeries. Another brought up the difficulty of obtaining the necessary continuing professional development (CPD) points to renew a license, as going to seminars and other forms of training may be rather expensive. People who can't afford these costs will have a hard time meeting their CPD obligations.

Reports of other difficulties in the delivery of clinical education include medical students' unwillingness to consult with patients, operating room congestion that endangers patients, and the prioritizing of private consultations for financial gain over instruction. Consequently, at graduation, doctors lack extensive hands-on experience with procedures. One possible way to fill these gaps may be by offering virtual reality training options. Patients in some areas were previously more willing to participate in educational roles.

However, many patients choose not to participate right away, which has raised concerns that medical graduates may not receive the same amount of hands-on experience due to increased reading levels. Virtual reality and other emerging technologies may be the key to closing this gap. Training scenarios that emphasize the quantity of procedures over the quality of information can promote less-than-ideal operating practices and lower overall training standards. The issue is exacerbated when competent individuals lack opportunities for postgraduate education or mentorship, potentially perpetuating ineffective methods and unprovoked errors. The members were concerned that if the instruction was not sufficiently clear, the public might mishandle their responsibilities, leading to ineffective practices or errors.

1.5.7 Realizing via Seeing: 360-Degree Visualization

This portion considers the potential benefits of using 360-degree standard television technology in surgical instruction and preparation. It highlights the advantages of this technology, including a dynamic and comprehensive view, increased engagement, improved accessibility, and effective comparisons between 360-degree videos and demonstrative imaging. Orthopaedic trainees have stressed the pertinence of 360-degree videos for improving procedural accuracy and have demonstrated their potential for knowledge building by sharing insights with peers.

However, there are disadvantages to ocular education alone, such as a need for hands-on training in performing complex procedures like laparotomies. Even the most precise visual models can overlook key details when compared to physical sketches. Despite these drawbacks, 360-degree standard videos are effective when used in conjunction with hands-on training as part of comprehensive surgical education.

The summary layout may include further information. Ensuring that healthcare professionals are executing their duties correctly is critically important, as mistakes made during training can lead to serious consequences throughout their careers. As an example, a physician performing complex procedures like tracheostomies needs a reliable way to develop their surgical judgement. One doctor observed that they could leverage their expertise with intubation, for instance. Medical experts in LMICs, who do not often handle these procedures, might find this very constructive. To assist physicians in regaining confidence and accuracy when performing new procedures, the idea of a library of convenient, video-recorded clinical techniques was developed. This information repository ensures that professionals are informed and prepared for all eventualities by encompassing the latest best practices.

1.5.8 Acceptability and Ease of Access

VR for medical instruction is not yet widely feasible in depressed- and middle-income countries, according to the study's participants. The most significant concern was the price, especially for the essentials like mobile phones and VR headsets, in addition to the need for a constant internet connection. Another major challenge was the unreliability of internet access, which was especially severe in remote locations. VR participants cited high data costs and frequent connectivity disruptions as significant challenges to VR training. Users stated pain and fatigue from continuous computer simulation usage, making necessary frequent breaks, despite the technology's ease of setup.

In contrast to the awkward and intermittent scheduling of conventional dispassionate lectures, participants also highlight that VR-enhanced training may advance public engagement, continuous learning, and networking for professional or personal gain. Concerns were raised about generational resistance, particularly among older physicians who may be hesitant to adopt new technologies. Younger doctors, however, mostly favoured virtual reality as a means to remain abreast of developments in their area and to facilitate ongoing education, irrespective of their location or time constraints.

1.6 DISCUSSION

Results from the mixed-methods research show that increasing global well-being with appropriate VR material for surgical instruction requires collaborative support networks between high-income countries (HICs) and LMICs. The study underscores a significant need for VR-based simulation in postgraduate surgical instruction across a range of educational and economic settings.

VR was a major attraction at the conference, even for those who were previously unfamiliar with the technology. Surveys taken after VR courses validated the technology's ease of use and suggested ways to incorporate it into existing medical curricula. Inadequate training programs owing to scarce resources, inconsistent training structures, and a lack of access to cutting-edge technology are just a few of the problems highlighted in the interviews as obstacles to clinical training in East Africa. Virtual reality can alleviate some of these problems. The real-world obstacles to adopting VR programs are highlighted in this research, including issues with cost, internet reliability, and combining virtual reality with clinical practice. VR can provide high-quality surgical training in settings with limited resources, and participants' positive reactions suggest that it is worth considering. The development of extended reality (XR) hubs and distribution of resources via mobile networks are key strategies for the expansion of this effort.

Virtual reality has the potential to revolutionize surgical education, but additional study with a group of controls and ongoing evaluation is needed to draw any firm conclusions about its long-term impact in training environments. The use of VR in medical education, particularly in underprivileged areas, is a significant step towards improved surgical training on a worldwide scale. This will allow for more accessible and inclusive learning experiences.

1.7 CONCLUSION

The first virtual reality training session for global surgery's emergency and critical procedures yielded very favourable qualitative and quantitative results. To facilitate the scalable distribution of material that is appropriate to local settings, the design approach highlights the significance of physicians, academics, educators, and technologists collaborating across LMICs and HICs. To fill the gaps in clinical education, there is a great need for virtual reality surgical training and its integration into current local educational programs. VRiMS has promised to hold more events to expand upon the knowledge gained. Qualitative research revealed many important issues, such as advantages, disadvantages, and future possibilities, that can guide VR-enhanced worldwide surgical education programs. Education is the main focus of this research, but there is growing evidence that next-generation technology and videoconferencing are transforming surgical instruction [17]. In conclusion, we show that postgraduate surgical teaching via remote VR has been successfully scaled up. This demonstrates the tremendous potential of XR technology to improve healthcare systems and encourage capacity-building globally.

REFERENCES

1. Hu, Kai-Chun, et al. "Impact of virtual reality anatomy training on ultrasound competency development: a randomized controlled trial." *PLoS One* 15.11 (2020): e0242731.
2. Mao, Randi Q., et al. "Immersive virtual reality for surgical training: a systematic review." *Journal of Surgical Research* 268 (2021): 40–58.
3. Lohre, Ryan, et al. "Improved complex skill acquisition by immersive virtual reality training: a randomized controlled trial." *JBJS* 102.6 (2020): e26.
4. William, S. Yi, et al. "A systematic review of immersive virtual reality for nontechnical skills training in surgery." *Journal of Surgical Education* 81.1 (2024): 25–36.
5. Angel-Urdinola, Diego F., Catalina Castillo-Castro, and Angela Hoyos. *A Meta-Analysis Assessing the Effects of Virtual Reality Training on Student Learning and Skills Development.* World Bank, 2021.
6. Chen, Xiuwen, et al. "Effect of virtual reality training to enhance laparoscopic assistance skills." *BMC Medical Education* 24.1 (2024): 29.
7. Kumar, T. Rajasanthosh, G. L., and S. Solomon Raj. "A framework of intelligent manufacturing process by integrating various function." In Deepa Jose, Preethi Nanjundan, Sanchita Paul, and Sachi Nandan Mohanty (eds) *AI-Driven IoT Systems for Industry 4.0.* CRC Press, 241–254.
8 Fazlollahi, Ali M., et al. "Effect of artificial intelligence tutoring vs expert instruction on learning simulated surgical skills among medical students: a randomized clinical trial." *JAMA Network Open* 5.2 (2022): e2149008.
9. Sivakumar, S., et al. "Scada energy management system under the distributed decimal of service attack using verification techniques by IIoT." *2023 International Conference on Artificial Intelligence and Knowledge Discovery in Concurrent Engineering (ICECONF).* IEEE, 2023.
10. Sommer, Guillermo Marcos, et al. "The role of virtual reality simulation in surgical training in the light of COVID-19 pandemic: visual-spatial ability as a predictor for improved surgical performance: a randomized trial." *Medicine* 100.50 (2021): e27844.
11. Barteit, Sandra, et al. "Augmented, mixed, and virtual reality-based head-mounted devices for medical education: systematic review." *JMIR Serious Games* 9.3 (2021): e29080.

12. Mewada, S., A. Saroliya, N. Chandramouli, T. Rajasanthosh Kumar, M. Lakshmi, S. Suma Christal Mary, and M. Jayakumar. "Research article smart diagnostic expert system for defect in forging process by using machine learning process." *System (In Section 4)* 19 (2022): 21.
13. Mewada, Shivlal, et al. "Smart diagnostic expert system for defect in forging process by using machine learning process." *Journal of Nanomaterials* 2022.1 (2022): 2567194.
14. Chen, Richard, et al. "A comprehensive review of robotic surgery curriculum and training for residents, fellows, and postgraduate surgical education." *Surgical Endoscopy* 34 (2020): 361–367.
15. Jiang, Haowen, et al. "Virtual reality in medical students' education: a scoping review." *JMIR Medical Education* 8.1 (2022): e34860.
16. Rathore, P. S., Ahuja, S., Burri, S. R., Khunteta, A., Baliyan, A., & Kumar, A. (2024). *Deep learning techniques for automation and industrial applications.* John Wiley & Sons, Inc.; Scrivener Publishing LLC.
17. Winkler-Schwartz, Alexander, et al. "Machine learning identification of surgical and operative factors associated with surgical expertise in virtual reality simulation." *JAMA Network Open* 2.8 (2019): e198363.
18. Huang, Ta-Ko, et al. "Augmented reality (AR) and virtual reality (VR) applied in dentistry." *The Kaohsiung Journal of Medical Sciences* 34.4 (2018): 243–248.
19. Alvarez-Lopez, Fernando, et al. "Use of a low-cost portable 3D virtual reality simulator for psychomotor skill training in minimally invasive surgery: task metrics and score validity." *JMIR Serious Games* 8.4 (2020): e19723.
20. Dhar, Poshmaal, et al. "Augmented reality in medical education: students' experiences and learning outcomes." *Medical Education Online* 26.1 (2021): 1953953.
21. Moll-Khosrawi, Parisa, et al. "Virtual reality as a teaching method for resuscitation training in undergraduate first-year medical students during COVID-19 pandemic: a randomised controlled trial." *BMC Medical Education* 22.1 (2022): 483.
22. Lungu, Abel J., et al. "A review on the applications of virtual reality, augmented reality and mixed reality in surgical simulation: an extension to different kinds of surgery." *Expert Review of Medical Devices* 18.1 (2021): 47–62.
23. Bayram, Sule Biyik, and Nurcan Caliskan. "The use of virtual reality simulations in nursing education, and patient safety." In Stanislaw P. Stawicki and Michael S. Firstenberg (eds) *Contemporary Topics in Patient Safety-Volume 1.* IntechOpen, 2020.
24. AlGerafi, Mohammed A. M., et al. "Unlocking the potential: a comprehensive evaluation of augmented reality and virtual reality in education." *Electronics* 12.18 (2023): 3953.
25. Mergen, Marvin, Norbert Graf, and Marcel Meyerheim. "Reviewing the current state of virtual reality integration in medical education-a scoping review." *BMC Medical Education* 24.1 (2024): 788.

CHAPTER 2

Immersive Technologies for Hazardous Material Response Training

Charanjeet Singh, Guna Sekhar Sajja, K. Suresh Kumar, Pramoda Patro, and M. Clement Joe Anand

2.1 INTRODUCTION

The medical field is just one of several that has seen virtual reality (VR) technology's meteoric rise in recent years [1]. Surgical training using virtual reality is one of the most exciting uses of VR in healthcare today. The popular notion is that hopeful surgeons should get their hands dirty working on cadavers, animals, or folk under close supervision while they learn something new [2–4]. That said, skill limitations pose significant challenges to each of these approaches. While cadaver-located education offers many benefits [5], it also has some disadvantages, such as the risk of infection, moral concerns, and a lack of suitable specimens [6–8]. Another popular area of research is based on the use of animals. However, due to physiological and anatomical dissimilarities between people and animals [9], this approach is not as effective for teaching processes that are specific to human surgery [10].

Furthermore, there are growing concerns about the ethical implications of utilizing animals in research [11]. Observational training, where undergraduates observe more experienced surgeons perform procedures [12], is not always sufficient and does not consistently provide residents with the chance to receive the hands-on experience they need to become competent surgeons [13].

DOI: 10.1201/9781003564904-2

Despite these barriers, medical instruction may benefit greatly from the use of computer-based simulation [14–16]. These simulators allow trainees to practice complex procedures repeatedly in a controlled, safe, and immersive setting, removing practical and ethical restraints [17]. These systems provide learners with valuable feedback by simulating real-life scenarios and incorporating patient-specific models [18].

Compared to other medical specialities, such as neurosurgery or laparoscopy, orthopaedic surgery has been relatively slow to adopt virtual training environments [19]. This is significant given the complexity of orthopaedic procedures, which require a detailed understanding of spatial relationships [20], mechanical forces, and the precise use of surgical instruments [21]. To address this need, this chapter analyzes the development of a VSE specifically designed for the orthopaedic procedure known as the Less Invasive Stabilization System (LISS) plating [22–24]. A modern technique for fixing fractures, the LISS plating method emphasizes minimizing damage to soft tissues while ensuring mechanical stability [25]. Virtual reality training is particularly well-suited to the LISS method because of its complexity and the high level of precision it requires [26]. Using advanced computer simulation technology [27], the VSE method replicates a surgical process with the same tools and components used in actual operations [28]. By following a virtual physician's step-by-step commands, scholars may practice the skills, techniques, and decision-making that are essential for actual surgical procedures [29]. The training experience is enhanced with accompanying features such as haptic feedback, visual realism, and real-time error detection [30], which make it more engaging and effective.

Orthopaedic medical procedures can benefit from these VR technologies in three ways: improved training outcomes, less reliance on conventional methods, and better patient care. This method aligns with current trends in medical education that stress technology-enhanced learning and utilizing evidence-based processes. Orthopaedic surgery can benefit from VR technologies in three key ways: improved training outcomes, reduced dependence on traditional teaching methods, and enhanced patient care.

2.2 LITERATURE REVIEW

This section provides a brief overview of the chapter on virtual reality in orthopaedic surgery. It summarizes the current state of VR applications in orthopaedic surgery and discusses the difficulties that have emerged.

Several research groups have developed VR simulators to aid in orthopaedic surgery procedures. To facilitate the development process's planning and execution, Cecil and Pirela-Cruz created an information model for virtual microsurgery.

Various researchers have explored different approaches to surgical planning in the treatment of fractures and other related ailments. While working on a virtual surgical simulator, Ruthenbeck and Reynolds provided a concise description of the many software tools needed for the project. Wolfson et al. reviewed traditional surgical training methods and the function and influence of virtual reality surgical simulations on the evolution of surgical education. Researchers also have looked at haptic technology for use in surgical simulation systems, particularly in programs designed for creating surgical models.

There are several gaps. When compared to other areas of surgery, orthopaedics is notoriously slow to adopt and implement virtual reality. It is necessary to create VR simulations to teach residents how to handle surgical operations involving fractures, as most of these simulators have concentrated on arthroscopic treatments. No previous study has dealt with the topic of LISS plating surgery, which is the focus of this chapter's research strategy.

The development of an information-centric foundation is an essential first step in designing and building VR-based simulations, although this area has received little attention in previous studies. This study's methodology suggests using information modelling methodologies, which might provide a systematic foundation for the development of such VSEs.

2.3 MEDICAL HISTORY OF SURGERY

The scope of the virtual surgical environment is restricted to the orthopaedic procedure known as less invasive stabilization system surgery, which is used to repair femur bone fractures. There are many stages to the LISS plating–based operation (Figure 2.1). The first step is the preoperative planning, which includes choosing the right implants for the identified fracture. After that, the surgeon will try to reduce the fracture. Utilizing an insertion guide, the LISS plate is placed in its correct position after the reduction of the fracture. Finally comes the most crucial part of the procedure: screwing the LISS plate into place on the bone using multiple types of surgical screws.

When aligned correctly above the femur, the LISS plate separates from the insertion guide. After that, the surgical wounds are sealed (Figure 2.2).

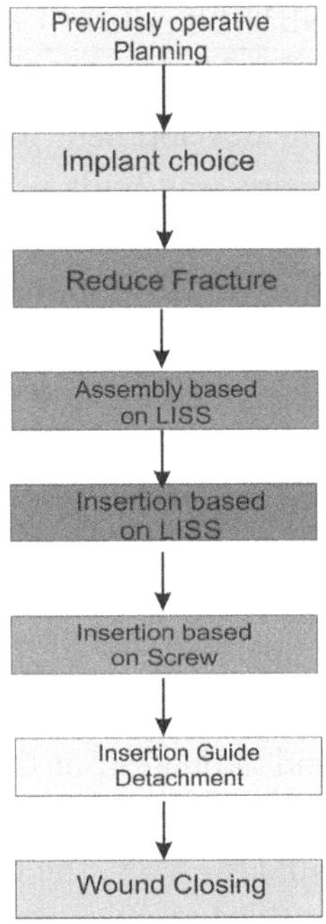

FIGURE 2.1 LISS plating–based operation stages.

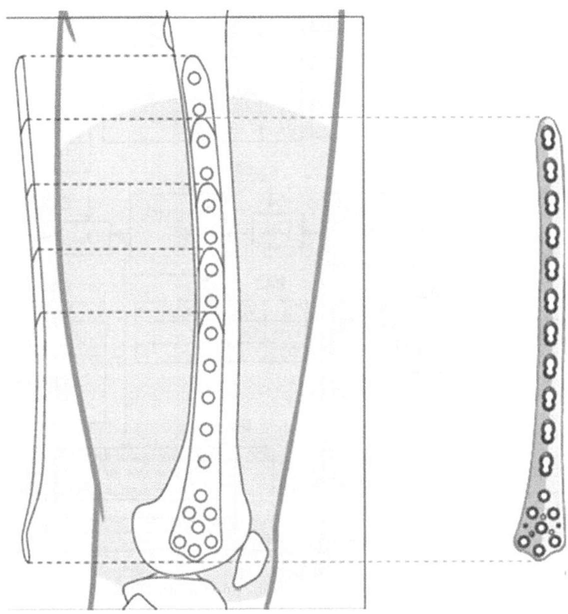

FIGURE 2.2 LISS plate separates from insertion guide.

2.4 DESIGN AND CONSTRUCTION OF THE VSE

Complex simulation environments built utilizing information modelling approaches are a recent development for many engineering applications. The VSE in this work was built using engineering Enterprise Modelling Language (eEML), an engineering enterprise modelling language. Information modelling makes use of a wide variety of modelling languages and methodologies, such as IDEF, unified modelling language (UML), and business process modelling language (BPML), among others.

The suggested technique is flexible enough to accommodate any modelling language. Since we have experience with HTML for the creation of VR-based software systems across a variety of fields and the analysis of data exchange activities in previous simulation-based projects, we are using it to construct VSE.

Figure 2.3 is an overview of the UML model that was used to outline the design, construction, and validation of the virtual surgical environment. A multiple-disciplinary team of surgeons, IT specialists, and engineers collaborated to build the VSE. The UML model offers a systematic basis for the VSE's design and construction.

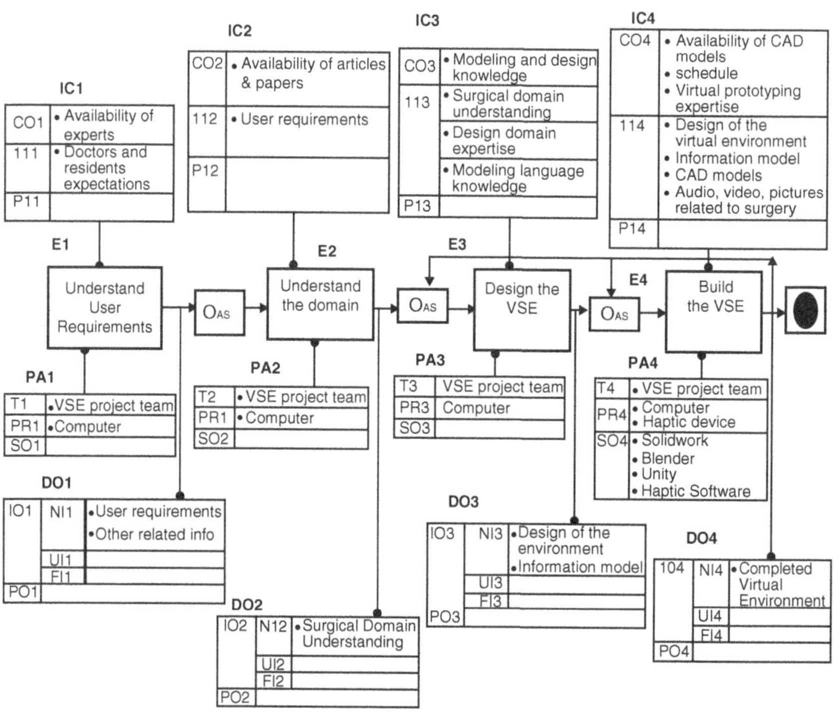

FIGURE 2.3 Overview of the UML method.

Entities and characteristics that are functional and necessary for the tasks at hand make up the UML model. E1 stands for "understand user requirements" while all the other entities represent different functional tasks. A collection of informational characteristics linked to each activity criteria that influence (IC), agents that perform (PA), and objects that decide (DO) are recognized. Some ways to classify the IC are by the types of inputs they include, such as physical, informational, and constraint-related factors (Figure 2.4). Team, physical, and software resources are the subcategories of PA. The decision objects include both physical and informational outputs.

The five stages of the VSE construction process are detailed as follows.

1. Gaining insight into user needs and preferences is the primary goal of task E1.
2. Reading books, articles, viewing films, etc., pertaining to the surgical realm is the major emphasis of E2.
3. Developing the architecture of the VSE, including determining which modules to use and how to best use them, is the responsibility of the E3 team.
4. In the fourth unit, participants will learn how to construct the VSE utilizing a variety of VR software and hardware.
5. The next step is to test the created VSE with seasoned surgeons and residents to ensure its accuracy.

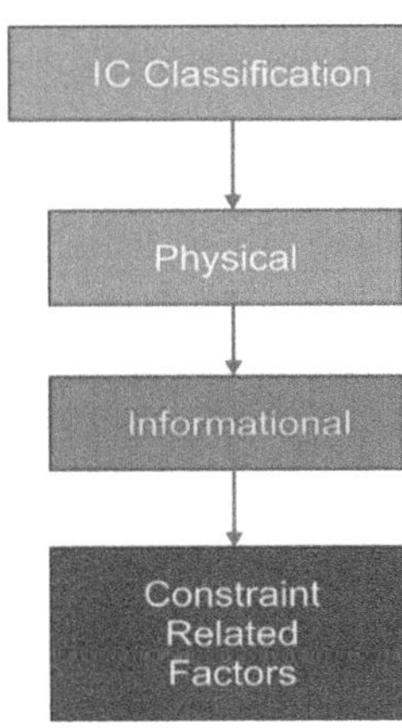

FIGURE 2.4 IC classificational ways.

All of the environments, haptic and otherwise, were created with the help of the Unity 3DTM game engine. Programs related to applications built in C# and JavaScript were used to construct the simulation environment.

2.5 STRUCTURE OF THE SYSTEM

A review of the essential components follows the visual representation of the VSE's design in Figure 2.5.

2.5.1 Structure of the System

Resident competency in the following surgical procedures is made possible by the training modules: Fracture reduction, LISS plate assembly. Step one involves inserting the LISS plate into the bone, step two involves placing and screwing the plate into place, and step three involves removing the screws. Figure 2.6 shows an overview of the VSE, which employs avatars to facilitate interactions as well. The position training module is the only one described here to keep things brief.

Residents will learn how to properly place the LISS plate for the patient's femur and surgical implants in the positional training module (Figure 2.7). Residents may learn the proper placement of the LISS plate for the skeleton and artificial prosthetics. Figure 2.7 shows that when the device is in the right place, an indicator glows blue. Residents may practice this vital

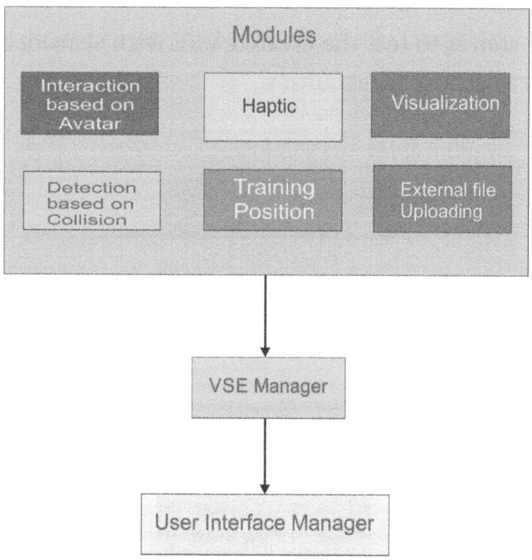

FIGURE 2.5 Visual representation of the VSE's design.

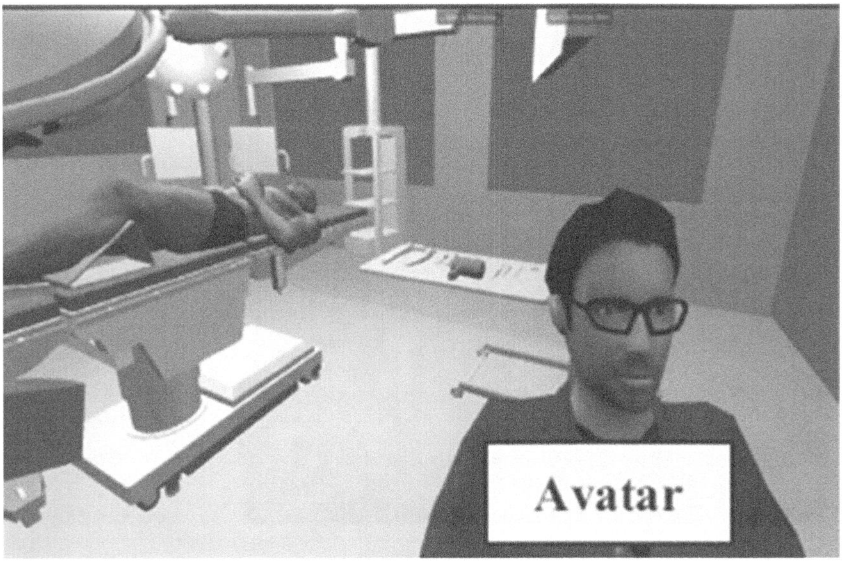

FIGURE 2.6 Overview of the VSE.

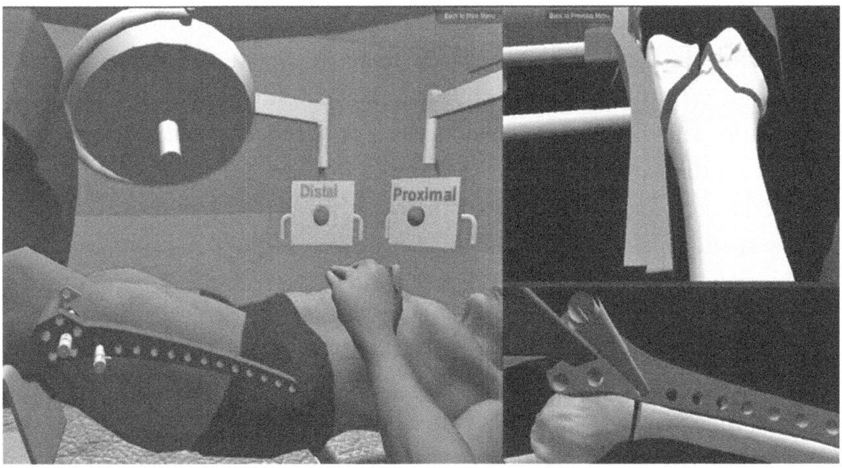

FIGURE 2.7 Positional training module.

activity interactively by placing the plate in the precise location and orientation. If they exceed the allowed limit, the indicator flashes green.

Figure 2.8 shows how to utilize a haptic interface—made possible by the Geomagic Touch™—to try out various phases in the LISS plate assembly process. By connecting with medical trainees in diverse places, a master surgeon may provide interactive training using the VSE. This is made

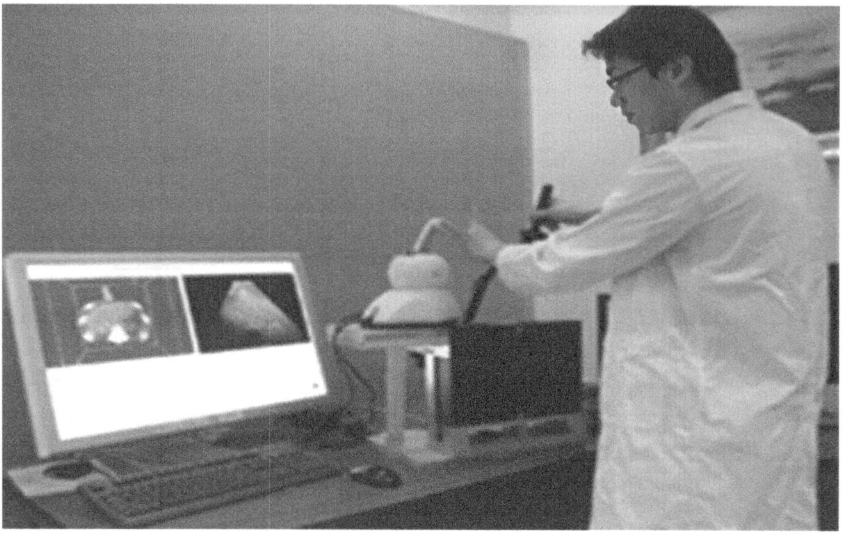

FIGURE 2.8 Haptic interface device with user.

possible through initiatives like GENI (geni.net) efforts and Next Generation Internet frameworks. By using these frameworks, complex applications in fields like healthcare will be able to transmit data at gigabit rates with minimal latency. The feasibility and advantages of remote collaboration and VSE-based instruction utilizing the GENI framework images are displayed in Figure 2.9a and b.

The latency data and bandwidth traffic measured between two GENI nodes at the same location for over 10 hours add up. All measurements were conducted using GENI Desktop, and ICMP ping was used to quantify network latency. The delay remains consistently below 1 millisecond, as is evident. The network traffic is enormous even with two nodes, which brings attention to the need for next-generation Internet with increased bandwidth capacity.

2.6 VALIDATION

Eleven orthopaedic residents from the Texas Technological University Health Science Centre in El Paso, Texas, performed a predetermined set of tasks to evaluate the Virtual Surgical Environment.

The first step in the validation process was a pre-test designed to gauge the residents' familiarity with the LISS plating procedure and their level of knowledge and competence in this area. To provide a baseline from which to measure future progress, this pre-test was essential.

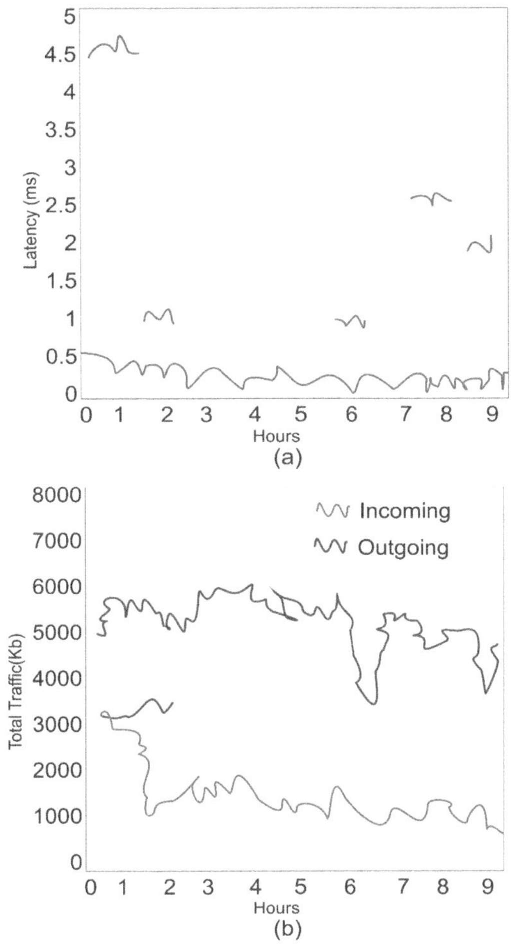

FIGURE 2.9 (a) Latency and (b) traffic.

After the initial trial, the residents used the VSE, an interactive and collaborative platform that provided comprehensive instruction on the LISS surgical procedure. By actively engaging in the process, participants were able to learn new aspects of the procedure in a controlled environment. Every member was required to take a post-test after finishing their VSE training in consideration of gauging using what much they had well-informed. Impressively, eight of the 11 residents showed solid progress in their understanding of and ability to complete the activity of the LISS surgical procedure. In comparison to common knowledge approaches, this augmentation shows the VSE's effectiveness as a training tool and its potential to improve education and skill development.

Ultimately, the results show that VSE training is a beneficial addition to medical school, contributing to a more effective approach to developing surgical ability. However, further validation studies are ongoing and will determine the impact of immersive simulation environments with haptic feedback compared to those without.

2.7 DISCUSSION

To improve surgical training and skill acquisition for residents, scientists focused on the development and design of a virtual reality–based surgical environment. The design process was extensively documented, highlightung how cutting-edge technologies were integrateded to create a dynamic and engaging lecture room background. In this study, we validated the VSE and established that it considerably enhanced surgical residents' educational outcomes by allowing them to practice and perfect surgical techniques in a reliable, simulated environment. Using Next Generation Internet technologies, researchers demonstrated that surgeons and residents from different parts of the country can collaborate in real time as enabled by the US Ignite and GENI initiatives.

This feature highlights the capability of the VSE to promote education via cooperation and inclusivity, even when users are geographically separated. The inclusion of cloud computing and high-speed networks further enabled this remote training model by ensuring smooth, real-time interaction.

2.8 CONCLUSION

Creating and utilizing the Virtual Reality Surgical Environment is a significant advancement in medical training and instruction. The VSE leverages cutting-edge computer simulation (VR) and Internet technologies to address major challenges in traditional surgical education, including limited resources, high-risk exposure, and geographical constraints. According to the validation study's findings, the VSE favourably raised surgical residents' technical skilfulness and confidence. Furthermore, the integration of next-generation Internet technologies through US Ignite and GENI programs shows the potential for collaborative, adaptable, and remote instructional platforms in the medical field. Future enhancements to the VSE include more complex surgical scenarios, AI-driven feedback systems, and support for interdisciplinary medical teams. This new method prepares future generations of surgeons to thrive in a dynamic healthcare environment by laying the foundation for a new era of medical education.

REFERENCES

1. Babalola, Akinloluwa, et al. "Applications of immersive technologies for occupational safety and health training and education: a systematic review." *Safety Science* 166 (2023): 106214.
2. Lee, J.S.A., et al. "Hazardous and toxic material decontamination facility training in virtual reality." *Electronics* 13.2 (2024): 465.
3. Jain, Avni. "Examining the use of virtual reality (VR) technology in health and safety training within hazardous work environments: a scoping review." (Doctoral dissertation, Auckland University of Technology). (2024).
4. Chen, Hao-Yang, Pey-Yune Hu, and Lien-Shang Wu. "Application of the Immersive Virtual Training: The First Immersive Simulation Cave System to the First Responder Training in Taiwan." *International Conference on Kansei Engineering & Emotion Research*. Singapore: Springer Nature Singapore, 2024.
5. Jamaludin, Nabila Farhana, et al. "Application of virtual reality (VR) in health, safety and environment subject for fire exit training module." *Journal of Advanced Research in Technology and Innovation Management* 12.1 (2024): 1–15.
6. Adel, A., and A. Elnogomi. "Enhancing oil and gas field HSE training through virtual reality." *Mediterranean Offshore Conference*. SPE, 2024.
7. Kumar, T.R., G. Laxmaiah, and S. Solomon Raj. "A framework of intelligent manufacturing process by integrating various function." In: T.R. Kumar, G. Laxmaiah, S.S. Raj, eds. *AI-Driven IoT Systems for Industry 4.0*. CRC Press. 241–254.
8. Muda, Ahmad Syazani, et al. "Advancing safety in the oil and gas infrastructure via virtual reality technology: a comprehensive exploration of hazard simulation and visualisations." *International Journal of Integrated Engineering* 16.9 (2024): 156–170.
9. Hazela, Bramah, et al. "Machine learning: supervised algorithms to determine the defect in high-precision foundry operation." *Journal of Nanomaterials* 2022.1 (2022): 1732441.
10. Faiz, Tauqeer, et al. "A scoping review on hazard recognition and prevention using augmented and virtual reality." *Computers* 13.12 (2024): 307.
11. Xu, Sheng, et al. "VR-based technologies: improving safety training effectiveness for a heterogeneous workforce from a physiological perspective." *Journal of Management in Engineering* 40.5 (2024): 04024032.
12. Dhotre, V.A., H. Mohammad, P.K. Pathak, A. Shrivastava and T.R. Kumar. "Big data analytics using map reduce for education system." *Linguistica Antverpiensia* 1 (2021): 3130–3138.
13. Luo, Yuan, et al. "Improving well control response ability via virtual reality technology." *Abu Dhabi International Petroleum Exhibition and Conference*. SPE, 2024.
14. Sariişik, Gencay. "The role of virtual reality technology in occupational safety training: applications and effects in the mining industry." *Research and Findings in Engineering Sciences* 2024 (2024): 153.
15. Berthiaume, Maxine, et al. "Evaluation of a virtual reality training tool for firefighters responding to transportation incidents with dangerous goods." *Education and Information Technologies* (2024): 1–39.

16. Sudiarno, Adithya, et al. "Investigating the future study area on VR technology implementation in safety training: a systematic literature review." *Journal of Safety Science and Resilience* 5 (2024): 235–248.
17. Yrjo, Tavion T., et al. "Enhancing risk assessment skills in hazardous environments: priming with a serious game approach." *Safety Science* 172 (2024): 106402.
18. Shayesteh, Shayan, et al. "Human-robot teaming in construction: evaluative safety training through the integration of immersive technologies and wearable physiological sensing." *Safety Science* 159 (2023): 106019.
19. Gong, Peizhen, et al. "Applications and effectiveness of augmented reality in safety training: a systematic literature review and meta-analysis." *Safety Science* 178 (2024): 106624.
20. Bao, Lan, et al. "Cross-platform virtual reality for real-time construction safety training using immersive web and industry foundation classes." *Automation in Construction* 143 (2022): 104565.
21. Shinde, Yugandhar. "Multi-modal personalized safety training to improve worker hazard identification performance." (MS thesis, Purdue University), 2023.
22. Haj-Bolouri, Amir. "Safe spaces for immersive safety training in virtual reality: a phenomenological conceptualization." *The International Journal of Virtual Reality* 24.1 (2024): 1–22.
23. Lyu, Jieyin, et al. "Intelligent-technology-empowered active emergency command strategy for urban hazardous chemical disaster management." *Sustainability* 15.19 (2023): 14369.
24. Spina, Sara. "Tools based on immersive technologies for supporting decision making to achieve sustainability and resilience in small and medium enterprises." (BS thesis, Universitat Politècnica de Catalunya), 2024.
25. Rai, M., Kumar, S., & Rathore, P. S. (2024). A systematic review of innovations for real-time image security in IoT applications using machine learning and blockchain. *Journal of Intelligent Manufacturing*, 1–20.
26. Alene, Gebray Habtu. "A novel framework for raising landslide risk awareness using immersive technology." (Doctoral thesis, NTNU). (2024). https://hdl.handle.net/11250/3157369
27. Aurelia, Sagaya. *Immersive Technologies: Navigating the Impacts, Challenges, and Opportunities*. CRC Press, 2024.
28. Pitsikalis, Stavros, et al. "Educational design guidelines for teaching with immersive technologies—updating learning outcomes of the European Qualification Framework." *Trends in Higher Education* 3.4 (2024): 1091–1108.
29. Blackler, Alethea, et al. "Supporting disaster preparedness through user-centred interaction design in immersive environments." In A. Blackler, N. Helsby-Clark, M.J. Ostwald, M. Foth (eds.), *Climate Disaster Preparedness: Reimagining Extreme Events through Art and Technology*. Cham: Springer Nature Switzerland, 2024. 123–136.
30. Dewan, Mohammud Hanif, et al. "Immersive and non-immersive simulators for the education and training in maritime domain—a review." *Journal of Marine Science and Engineering* 11.1 (2023): 147.

CHAPTER 3

Disaster Secure Simulation by Virtual Reality to Reduce the Rescue Operation

Lakshminarayana Reddy Kothapalli Sondinti, Ravi Kumar Vankayalapati, P.R. Sudha Rani, and R. Senthamil Selvan

3.1 INTRODUCTION

The standard method for treating brain tumours is the surgical removal of the tumour. To remove the tumour, doctors make an incision in the skull and then use a scalpel to remove the visible parts of the tumour [1, 2]. Surgeons are required to complete extensive neurosurgical training to learn techniques to administer treatments of varied degrees of complexity, ensuring that their patients always get high-quality results [3]. On the other hand, the time and money needed for conventional training methods are substantial. Consequently, doctors are looking for ways to teach their surgical staff more effectively and inexpensively, and computerized surgical training is one possible solution [4].

Surgeons use magnetic resonance (MR) pictures taken before surgery to help them find the growth they want to remove [5–8]. It does not, however, have the 3D anatomical direction of the surrounding tissues that this 2D image-based method does. Furthermore, users have to keep switching

DOI: 10.1201/9781003564904-3

between the surgery field and the MR pictures, which makes the process harder and less accurate [9]. Augmented reality (AR) can greatly improve doctors' visual experience by fusing image technologies with real objects and giving users a three-dimensional spatial association. Consequently, by using augmented reality in neurosurgical management, physicians can simultaneously see the actual operating environment and the concealed anatomical images [10–12]. This would make surgery much more successful and effective.

Some neurosurgical simulators have been verified for use in actual neurosurgery as their adoption in neurosurgery becomes increasingly common [13]. Designed to replicate neurosurgery operations including brain tumour removal, endoscope nasal navigation, and ventriculostomy, NeuroTouch is a VR simulator. Simple physical events, like brain deformation as well as tissue loss, are simulated using the finite element method [14–16]. The computer can check how much tissue is being removed and how much blood is being lost in simulated surgeries using physical modelling [17]. They built a whole virtual world where complicated bodily patterns, patient-specific anatomy, and detailed performance measures can be recreated. VR-based training system users, on the other hand, are fully involved in the virtual world and can forget they are in reality because of the way visualization works [18, 19]. While compared to VR systems, AR systems are more realistic because they add elements of the virtual setting into the way a person observes the real world. Additionally, AR systems' "see-through" display mode allows users to manipulate the surgical simulator and the actual surgical field more easily, as well as synchronize their vision with the procedure [20]. Furthermore, two shafts in a box are often used to represent the surgical instruments in the VR-based simulator. Compared to actual surgery, this is significantly different. Real and virtual items may be combined using stereo-tracking technology in an AR-based simulator [21–23].

This enhances both the ability to accurately see the operating area and fully immerse oneself in the surgical environment. To determine whether an AR technique is appropriate for guiding neurosurgery, a neurosurgery simulator is utilized, which has many advantages for users, such as gaining experience without putting patients at risk, learning from mistakes, and practising complicated cases [24, 25]. An augmented reality neurosurgery training simulator is created to help surgeons gain the knowledge to manipulate brain tumour resections more intuitively and naturally, allowing for more immersive and realistic neurosurgery training. The approach uses deep Voxelwise Residual Nets (VoxResNet) to accurately segment and rebuild 3D personalized brain anatomy. By methodically locating markers and calibrating the stereo monitoring device and HoloLens, the 3D virtual brains can be perfectly registered with the 3D-printed skull. This makes it possible to superimpose a virtual brain on top of a real skull in a holographic display.

3.2 METHODS

This research presents haptic-interaction, AR-guided neurosurgical training simulators for brain tumour excision operations using Microsoft HoloLens and Geomagic Touch. To make neurosurgery operations easier, more accurate, and more efficient, researchers eventually want to use AR guidance in neurosurgical training and help end-users approach the marked tumours precisely. A bimanual haptic interface with a holographic, VR spatial data visualization, and patient-specific brain anatomy reconstructions make up the system. An advanced perspective of the proposed system is shown in Figure 3.1.

3.2.1 Reconstruction of the Patient's Anatomy

The accuracy of neurosurgical modelling is heavily influenced by anatomical reconstruction. So, to develop the AR-based guide for neurosurgery, it is first necessary to accurately reconstruct a 3D line representation of the brain of a particular patient that includes the brain tissue, blood vessels, and tumours. An MRI is the preferred imaging modality for diagnosing brain abnormalities. However, it remains challenging to precisely separate the brain structures as well as tumours from MRI scans that show fine detail. To correctly segment the MRI of the brain, the open source VoxResNet is used in this study. Researchers further refine the resulting mesh utilizing a recently created bi-sane filtering method to reduce noise while preserving the essential anatomical features after segmentation. This process enables the reconstruction of a highly detailed, patient-specific virtual anatomical model, as shown in Figure 3.2.

3.2.2 Physical Interactions

To ensure realistic behavior of deformable bodies during the interactive progressive cutting process, precise contact modelling is essential in a surgical planning system. Interactions between surgical tools and tissue, as well as between different tissue layers, provide contact forces that function as limits within the dynamic model and cause mechanically accurate

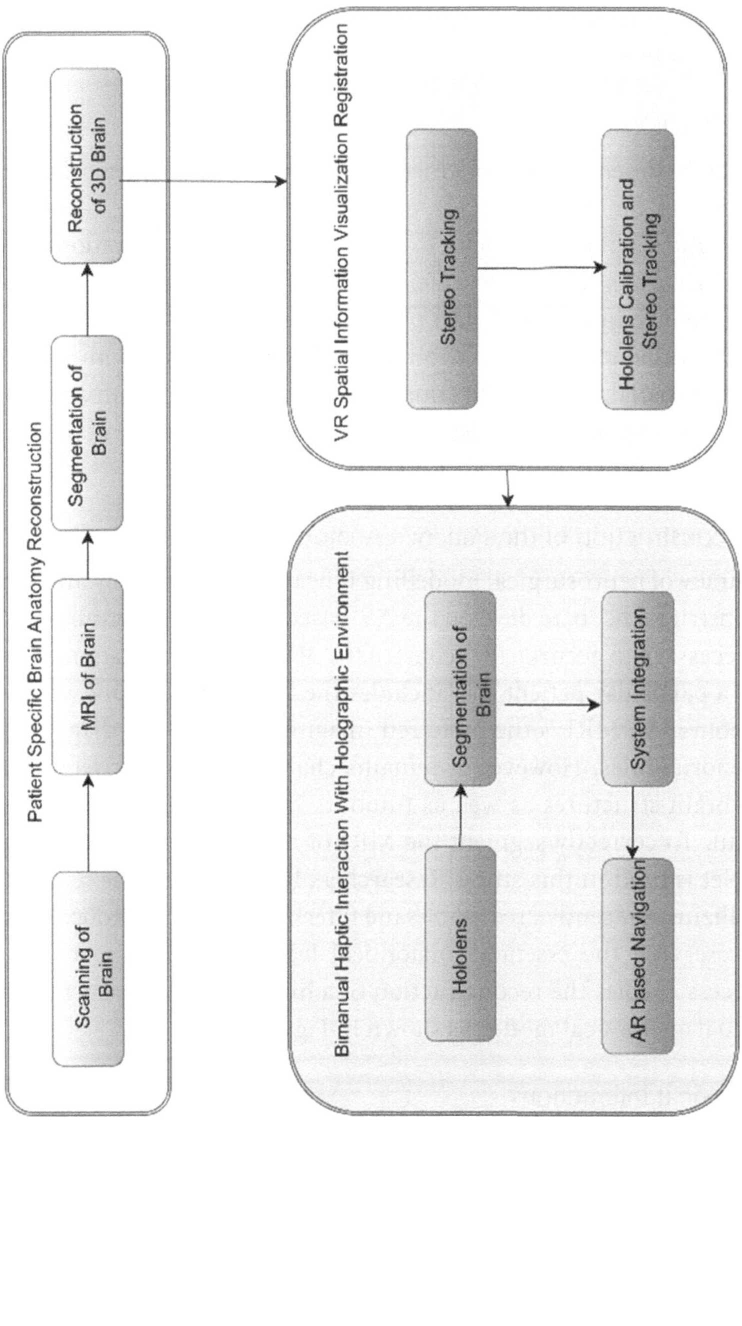

FIGURE 3.1 Schematic view of AR guidance.

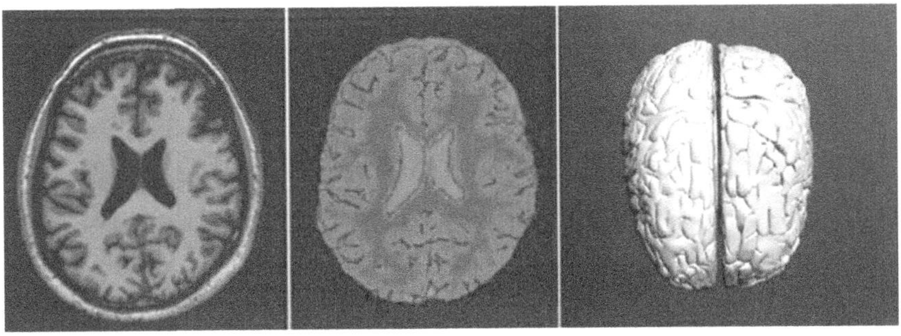

FIGURE 3.2 Segmentation of brain.

deformation responses. Both theoretically and numerically, frictional contact issues are fairly complex. Instead of the typical continuity feature that holds in solid mechanics, they are distinguished by a gap at the interface that is both geometric and material. As a result, contact questions are by their very nature non-linear, even non-smooth, characterized by constrained minimizations and variational prejudices. Using Coulomb's friction model and the Signorini condition in the composite lines model, the researcher can remedy the frictional interaction issues involved in both tool-tissue and tissue-tissue interactions during surgical training. The penalty method, which is represented as the contact force F_c, allows us to resolve the behavior of the finish and fabric contact.

$$F_c = k\delta\vec{n} \tag{3.1}$$

Here the interpretation is denoted by δ, $\vec{n}$ is the contact normal, which is the hypotenuse of the triangle where the contact point is placed and $k = \frac{1}{h^2}M + \frac{1}{h}D + K$.

3.2.3 Cut and Deform with a Biomechanical Model

Trauma, laceration, and haemorrhage to the brain are all physical events involved in brain tumour removal manoeuvres. To create a realistic virtual surgical environment, it is crucial to accurately simulate these operations. The brain's biomechanical deformability will be experienced due to the complexity of its various structures. To simulate brain deformation, a soft tissue model based on mass-spring systems is implemented. The model accurately describes the biomechanical behaviour of the brain tumours and vasculature by simulating the interactions between multiple types of structures, each with its own unique set of material properties.

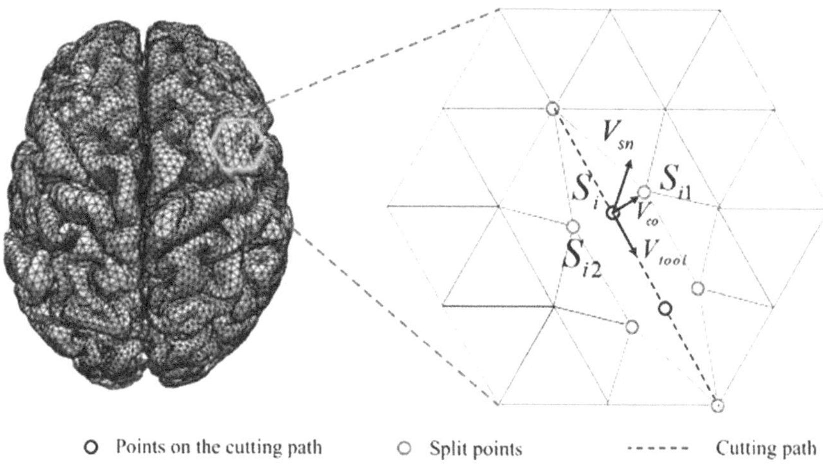

FIGURE 3.3 Methods of cutting.

A system of mass points and a network of springs were used to separate the soft tissue. For objects with complex material values like viscoelasticity and nonlinearity, the mass-spring model works well. An equation that describes the behavior of a mass-spring system is typically expressed as:

$$Mx^2(t) + Dx(t) + Kx = F \tag{3.2}$$

In this study, the researcher used the mass-spring model to simulate the relevant tissue deformation during the progressive cutting process. First, identify the collision points on the mesh structure prior to the incision. Next, the brain's elastic properties such as elastin and tau are updated using the mass-spring model. Lastly, when the contact force exceeds a predefined threshold, divide the cutting path into two sections by duplicating each affected point into two corresponding nodes.

The bulk point in the cutting route, S_i, is duplicated and displaced to two opposite sides of the path, creating two new points, S_{i1} and S_{i2}, as shown in Figure 3.3. The original mass point S_i is then removed because the displacement route is perpendicular to the cutting path. It is possible to determine the new connections between all polygon edges and their duplicate points S_{i1} and S_{i2} by removing the point S_i and then connecting them to:

$$S_{i1} = S_i + \frac{W}{2} V_{co}, S_{i2} = S_i - \frac{W}{2} V_{co} \tag{3.3}$$

$$V_{co} = \frac{1}{V_{tool} * V_{sn}} V_{tool} \times V_{sn} \tag{3.4}$$

3.2.4 Registration for the Display of Spatial Information in Virtual Reality

Registration of the virtual item, in reality, is necessary for AR-based guiding to work properly. Holographic brain surgery is put over top of a 3D-printed head using Microsoft HoloLens. As if they were operating, the "see-through" mode lets the user easily get close to the tumour of interest. On both the physical model and the virtual head model, several non-coplanar points are selected and marked. A standardization of the HoloLens within the NDI tracking of the stereo scheme is needed before the display registration can happen. The following steps are followed:

First Step: After positioning the NDI method marker on the HoloLens, determine its positioning concerning the NDI vertical course, then determine the angle α_{NDI} between the two.

Second Step: To determine the angle α_{H} between the Y axis and the NDI downward, it is necessary to locate the Y direction using the HoloLens coordinate technique. Step two involves determining the angle $(\alpha_{\text{H}} - \alpha_{\text{NDI}})$ that separates the HoloLens's position from its coordinate system.

Third Step: In the HoloLens, a virtual circle is placed, andthe origin of the HoloLens' coordinate system is aligned with it. When the virtual circle is positioned at the NDI coordinate system's origin, the HoloLens reference frames and NDI reference frames origins are at the same location. To align the two coordinate systems,the angular offset between their respective X and Y axes must therefore be measured. $T(\alpha_{\text{H}} - \alpha_{\text{NDI}})$ can calculate the measurement matrix.

Fourth Step: It is practicable to get the equivalent HoloLens position C from an NDI position C by using the formula $C = T(\alpha_{\text{H}} - \alpha_{\text{NDI}}) \times C_s$.

By following the locations of the skull model, this may be used to both register and place the virtual head onto a real scene using feature points after the HoloLens has been calibrated using the NDI stereoscopic tracking system.

3.2.5 Haptic Interaction between Two Users in a Holographic Setting

Using two Geomagic Touch devices, the Bimanual Haptic Augmented Interactions provides first-rate haptic and visual assistance. Two tactile devices are interconnected using the OpenHaptic toolbox that offers them both access and control, and the system is developed using Unity3D. The UNET unit in Unity3D designates the desktop as the server and the HoloLens as the client. The subsequent stage involves the system calculating the haptic forces, coordinating the placement and orientation of the virtual surgical instruments, and monitoring the motions of the two Geomagic Touch devices. Next, the penalty method is used to figure out the tactile forces that are created when simulated instruments as well as virtual brains collide with the Signorini condition. On the other hand, the stiffness ratio among the items that are touching or entering each other decides which penalty to use. It is recommended that the update rate for haptic feedback be 1000 Hz, while the rate for visible feedback should be between 25 and 60 Hz.

To constitute the haptic response, the researcher provides the multirate pattern. In greater detail, the mass-spring model is used to calculate the significant deformation of brain's soft tissue, helping to resolve the response forces induced by tool-tissue interaction. The project aims to enhance haptic feedback, making it more natural and realistic by using a B-spline continuous interpolation method to enhance the progression of force feedback. As shown in Figure 3.4, the developed neurosurgery training simulator combines bi-manual haptic response.

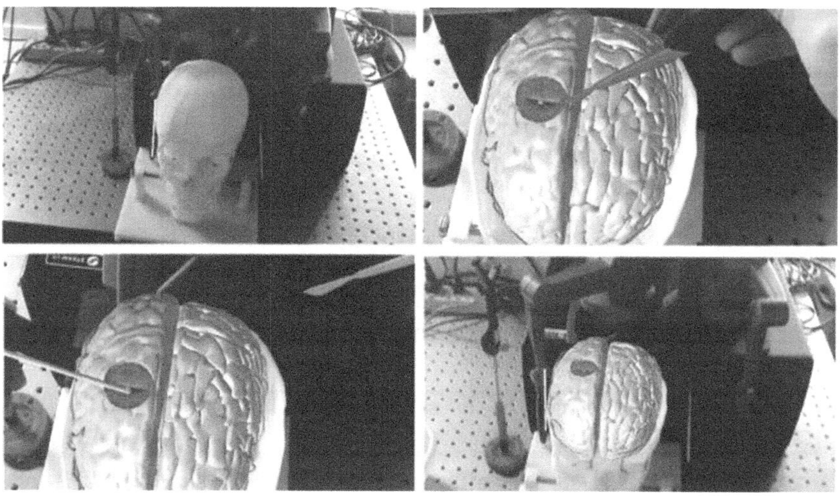

FIGURE 3.4 Neurosurgery assistance by AR.

3.3 RESULTS

A user study is done to check both the content and face validity of the AR-based neurosurgical training model. Its performance is also evaluated.

3.3.1 Virtual Neurosurgery

In order to evaluate the AR guidance mode, the surgical operation is done with AR guidance. The brain's 3D shape mesh is made up of 29,985 triangles and 14,734 points, thanks to the brain structure modelling method. It is much easier to remove a brain tumour when A 3D-printed skull matches the rebuilt brain structure. This enables us to observe the brain's hidden structures, including blood vessels, brain soft tissue, and target tumours.

Also, our simulator's "see-through" monitor lets users engage naturally, which helps them coordinate their vision as well as operation, which makes brain tumour removal more accurate.

3.3.2 Validation of Reliability

To assess the accuracy of AR control, researchers also created a precise 3D-printed model and skull for the accuracy validation experiment. A verification experiment is shown in Figure 3.5. Using the customized CT/MR scans, a virtual skull is created. In order to measure the distance inaccuracy and angle errors of the AR-based navigation, the 3D-printed template and skull were created with several markers that lay at a standard distance of great accuracy (0.1 mm).

This experiment evaluates all the steps involved in a typical augmented reality–based neurosurgery. These steps include registering the physical and virtual environments, tracking and positioning the surgical instruments, and performing the surgery itself. Before calibrating the placement

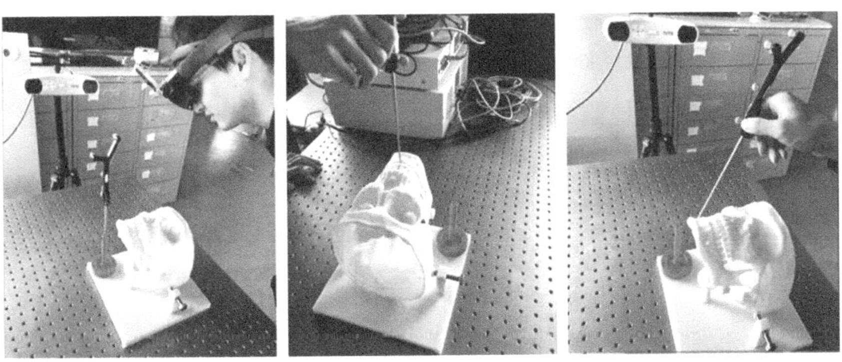

FIGURE 3.5 Verification of the accuracy of the surgical guidance system.

of surgery models, the researcher set a 3D-printed brain and reference model in the tracking area of the 3D monitoring and locating system. This was achieved by utilizing marks on both the 3D-printed brain and the virtual 3D brain model to register the templates. Researchers identified the marker positions on both the 3D-printed head and the virtual brain using the HoloLens to register settings in both real life and the virtual space. The next step was to verify that the 3D-printed brain and the virtual brain model are correctly aligned. Researchers further determined the relative positions of the reference markers utilizing both the tracking system and the virtual marks on the virtual skull. The distance error was then used to confirm that the system was working correctly. It's feasible to figure out the register mistake as follows: Let the marks in the 3D-printed skull along with the template be located in positions $C_1, C_2, \ldots, C_n$. This approach suggests that they are at positions $C'_1, C'_2, \ldots, C'_n$.

$$T_{\text{reg}} = \sqrt{\frac{\sum \| C_i - C_i' \|}{n}} \tag{3.5}$$

Here i take the values from 1 to n.

Ten feature points are chosen for the purpose of evaluating registration errors in the experiment. Table 3.1 shows the actual and registered locations of all feature points. The outcomes demonstrate that the suggested registration procedure achieves a mean target registration error of 2.12 mm.

TABLE 3.1 Statistics on AR Performance

Labels	Recorded Place (mm)	Original Place (mm)	Dislocation (mm)	Recorded Error (mm)
1	59.13, −83.20, −810.27	58.32, −82.98, −809.94	−0.82, 0.23, 0.34	0.91
2	55.54, −64.02, −808.88	55.26, −62.98, −809.54	−0.29, 1.03, −0.67	1.26
3	61.22, −41.73, −812.15	61.06, −41.91, −811.52	−0.17, −0.19, 0.64	0.68
4	61.81, −87.33, −836.87	58.53, −85.10, −837.64	−3.29, 2.24, −0.78	4.05
5	61.79, −41.04, −836.87	63.65, −39.86, −835.72	1.88, 0.19, 1.07	2.17
6	42.60, −122.14, −904.08	42.03, −66.91, −881.99	−0.58, 1.51, −0.85	1.82
7	85.03, −123.14, −905.08	85.01, −120.78, −903.76	−0.02, 2.37, 1.33	2.71

(Continued)

TABLE 3.1 (CONTINUED)

Labels	Recorded Place (mm)	Original Place (mm)	Dislocation (mm)	Recorded Error (mm)
8	45.64, −91.16, −895.15	44.73, −90.06, −896.06	−0.92, 1.11, −0.92	1.70
9	47.55, −44.33, −897.45	46.78, −43.39, −896.81	−0.78, 0.95, 0.65	1.38
10	34.65, −68.31, −908.26	36.42, −68.07, −908.81	1.78, −0.77, 1.26	2.31

3.3.3 Analysis of End-Users

For the AR-based neurosurgery training method, a handler study was set up to check its face and content validity. To find out how well the AR guide works and how much the simulation neurosurgery is like real neurosurgery, the questionnaire was made after talking with a neurosurgery expert. Ten people who hadn't done real neurosurgery were asked to take part. They had seen a training movie about neurosurgery and already knew about the surgical scene where the brain was deformed and cut. They also used surgical tools to cut muscle and fat on animals. For the AR setting, the "realistic" questions mostly look at how much the AR-based neurosurgical training model is like the real surgery presented in the teaching video. People ask how "realistic" virtual surgical tools and haptic operations are by comparing how they feel to real surgical instruments.

To explain the purpose and use of the AR-based neurosurgical training simulations, the researcher created a technical instruction document. The participants were allowed to manipulate the apparatus for ten minutes. One neurosurgical operation had to be completed six times by the volunteers. They had to locate the tumour within the brain tissue and perform the procedure to remove it. Participants were asked to fill out an online survey after the research to assess face and content validity. In response to comments, participants were asked to choose "agree," "neutral," or "disagree." To ensure that the claims made about the virtual and actual instruments' interactions with brain tissue were accurate, researchers asked participants to rate the following claims about the instruments' behaviour:

Question 1: The soft brain tissue of the AR world looked like the original.

Question 2: The growth in the brain material in the AR world looked like the original.

Question 3: The brain tissue and growth in the 3D-printed head that were based on AR were real.

Question 4: The head that was 3D made looked like the original.

Question 5: The soft tissue change in the brain in the AR world was like the original.

Question 6: It felt real to cut brain matter in the AR world.

Question 7: It felt real when the virtual surgery tools and brain matter touched each other.

Question 8: The way the brain cells and the growth interacted was believable.

Question 9: The mechanical device was placed correctly.

Question 10: It was correct for the virtual surgery tool and the mechanical device to register in real time.

Question 11: When the haptic device is used, it feels like the medical tools are used.

Question 12: The time lag between moving something and seeing a result was reasonable.

Question 13: The physical force feedback felt like original.

This questionnaire's face validity scores for all subjects are shown in Figure 3.6. On questions 1 through 3, subjects were asked to rate how realistic they thought it was to see brain soft tissue along with tumours in the AR world. Ninety-one per cent of them said "agree," which means they believed it was true. Question 4: Everyone agreed that the 3D-printed head looks real. Concerning questions 5–8 that looked at how brain soft tissue behaves physically and how it interacts in neurosurgery modelling, 81% of people said they "agree," 9% said they were "neutral," and 9% said they "disagree." Ten per cent of those who answered the questions about the AR-based navigation system's performance (Q9–Q13) said they "disagreed," while 9% said they "agreed." Seventy per cent said they "agreed," saying that the registration among the virtual surgical tool as well as the haptic device was real time and correct (Q10), while 20% said they were "neutral," and 10% said they "disagreed." It was confirmed by 71% of "agree" responses that using the haptic device felt like using medical tools

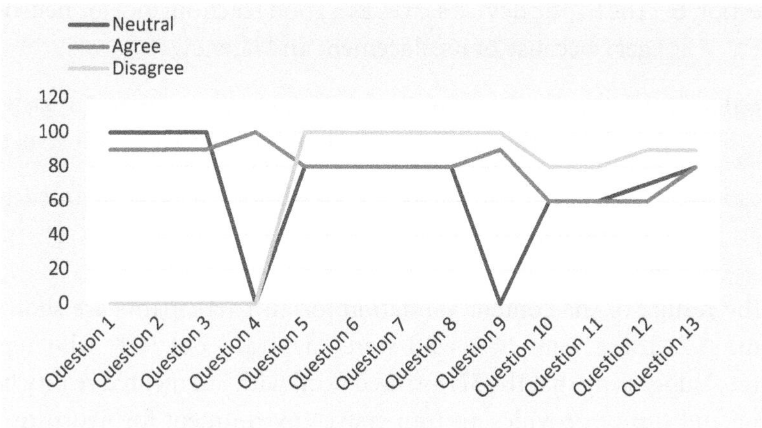

FIGURE 3.6 Outcomes of face evaluation.

(Q11); 10% of responses were "neutral," and 21% of responses were "disagree." There were 71% "agree" responses to question 12 about whether the delay between physical manipulation along visual reaction was realistic, 21% "neutral" responses, and 11% "disagree" responses. There were also 81% "agree" responses to question 13 about whether the haptic force feedback felt realistic, 10% "neutral" responses, and 10% "disagree" responses. The following statements were given to subjects as content evaluation questions to see how useful they thought the simulator was as a neurosurgery training tool and how well the virtual tasks were put together.

Question 1: With the use of augmented reality brain cells and a 3D-printed tumor, a neurosurgical training environment might be built.

Question 2: There is enough of the 3D-printed skull to make it a practical neurosurgical teaching aid.

Question 3: The distortion of brain tissue is sufficient to function as an effective neurosurgical teaching tool.

Question 4: There is enough cutting behaviour in the cerebral soft tissue to make it a practical neurosurgical teaching aid.

Question 5: The way the virtual surgical tool interacts with the brain tumor and soft tissue makes it a useful tool for neurosurgery instruction.

Question 6: The haptic device serves as a good teaching tool for neurosurgery because of its placement and latency.

Question 7: The haptic device and virtual surgical equipment register in real time, making it a useful tool for neurosurgery instruction.

Question 8: In general, the simulator serves as a helpful neurosurgical training aid.

The results of the content validation for all participants are shown in Figure 3.7. There were 10% who were "neutral," but 90% who replied "agree," suggesting that the 3D-printed skull with augmented reality brain tissue and tumor provides an immersive environment for neurosurgical training (Q1). Every participant unanimously responded in the affirmative when asked whether the 3D-printed skull will be used in surgical training (Q2). Seventy per cent of participants selected "agree" (Q3–Q4), suggesting that the simulation's cutting and deformation features are sufficient to make it a useful teaching tool for neurosurgery. Ten per cent stayed "neutral," and 10% disapproved of the concept. According to the results of Question 5, 60% of respondents "agree" that employing a virtual surgical tool in combination with brain soft tissue and tumors sufficiently prepares neurosurgical training, while 21% were "neutral" and 11% disagreed. Ninety-one per cent of respondents "agree" that the location and delay of the haptic device were sufficient for evaluating the performance of the augmented reality system, compared to 11% who were "neutral" (Q6). Ninety-one per cent of respondents said that they "agree" that the haptic device and virtual surgical tool are appropriately recorded in real time,

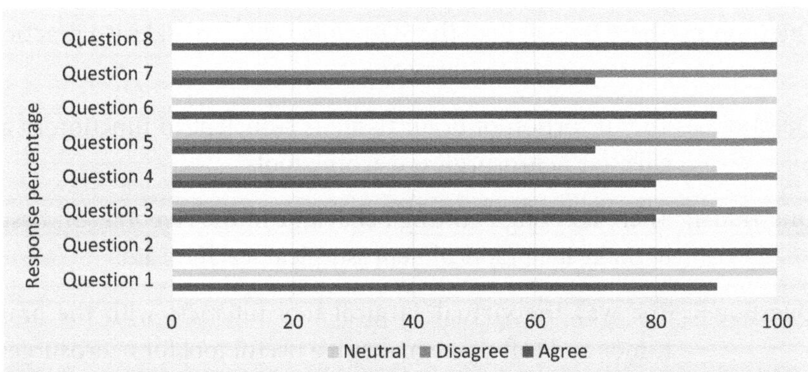

FIGURE 3.7 Outcome of content evaluation.

compared to 11% who "disagree" and 21% who were "neutral" (Q7). All participants responded "agree" to the statement that a simulator is a useful training tool in neurosurgery (Q8).

3.4 DISCUSSION

The most straightforward and efficient way to treat a variety of brain disorders is via neurosurgery, which is also one of the hardest procedures. In order to prevent harm to healthy tissues including blood vessels and peripheral nerves, surgeons must precisely resect the lesion. Accurate preoperative surgical planning and precise intraoperative lesion identification are critical to neurosurgical success.

Surgeons usually use the guide information from the MRI images taken before surgery to get close to the growth they want to remove. But there are two problems with the present way of instruction. First, the knowledge about preoperative advice is kept separate from the site during surgery. Surgeons have to move their eyes back and forth among the MRI images and the operating site on the patient in order to see where the tools are in relation to the patient's anatomy. This is not ideal because it can make it hard for them to focus. This will get in the way of the surgery and make guiding mistakes more likely. Second, it's hard for surgeons to figure out the guidance information on the 2D MRI images that are taken before surgery because they don't show the exact location of the surgical tools in 3D space. Because of this, doctors can't naturally understand how the surgical tool fits in relation to the patient's body in the operating room, which means that the current training method isn't good enough.

There are a few benefits of using AR for neurosurgical surgical training. Surgeons are able to precisely evaluate the relative location of various structures with the use of augmented reality, which supplies them with accurate, patient-specific anatomical structural information. Surgeons may easily find the optimal tumor access method with the help of precise anatomical depiction and quantitative assessment. As a result of associating the rebuilt anatomical structure with the surgical site, augmented reality allows surgeons to intuitively examine the inside structure, providing clear guiding information for doing the surgery. Neurosurgeons can practice real surgeries with the AR-based neurosurgical training model that was made. But there are some problems with the system that was developed. While the video image of neurosurgery is realistic, real neurosurgery has additional information, like how the blood flows and how the blood vessels pulse. To make a realistic surgery scene, the modeling of the AR world also needs work. For more accurate and immersive surgical direction, the AR world should include more realistic simulations of blood flow and vessel pulsatility, as well as better modeling effects.

3.5 CONCLUSIONS

This research explores the possibilities of using augmented reality technology for neurosurgery training. The developed neurosurgical training simulator can teach surgeons the fundamentals of the field in an extremely realistic and intuitive fashion, according to the results of the experiments. However, due to the nature of the registration issue and the simplicity of boundary conditions, the current study is limited to a simulated environment. In order to enable AR-based imaging of target areas in surgical navigation, researchers must eventually register with enough precision in a real-world clinical setting. Meanwhile, researchers are interested in refining the rendering effects and modeling the specifics of blood flow and vascular pulsatility. The further effort also includes extending to other guided operations.

REFERENCES

1. Itamiya, Tomoki. "Using virtual reality and augmented reality for enhancing school education." In Yildiz, A., Shaw, R. (eds) *Disaster and Climate Risk Education: Insights from Knowledge to Action*. Singapore: Springer Nature Singapore, 2024. 379–397.
2. Biswal, Anil Kumar, et al. "Mobile-based weather forecasting and visualization using augmented reality." In Samanta, D. (ed) *Designing and Developing Innovative Mobile Applications*. IGI Global, 2023. 125–137.
3. Dunleavy, Matt, Chris Dede, and Rebecca Mitchell. "Affordances and limitations of immersive participatory augmented reality simulations for teaching and learning." *Journal of Science Education and Technology* 18 (2009): 7–22.
4. Li, Xiao, et al. "A critical review of virtual and augmented reality (VR/AR) applications in construction safety." *Automation in Construction* 86 (2018): 150–162.
5. Rathore, P. S., S. Ahuja, S. R. Burri, A. Khunteta, A. Baliyan, & A. Kumar. (2024). *Deep learning techniques for automation and industrial applications*. John Wiley & Sons, Inc.; Scrivener Publishing LLC.
6. Vávra, Petr, et al. "Recent development of augmented reality in surgery: a review." *Journal of Healthcare Engineering* 2017.1 (2017): 4574172.
7. Singh, C., M. S. Srinivasa Rao, Y. M. Mahaboobjohn, B. Kotaiah, and T. Rajasanthosh Kumar. "Applied machine tool data condition to predictive smart maintenance by using artificial intelligence." In *International Conference on Emerging Technologies in Computer Engineering*, pp. 584–596. Cham: Springer International Publishing, 2022.

8. Klopfer, Eric, and Kurt Squire. "Environmental detectives—the development of an augmented reality platform for environmental simulations." *Educational Technology Research and Development* 56 (2008): 203–228.
9. Chi, Hung-Lin, Shih-Chung Kang, and Xiangyu Wang. "Research trends and opportunities of augmented reality applications in architecture, engineering, and construction." *Automation in Construction* 33 (2013): 116–122.
10. Van Krevelen, D. W. F., and R. Poelman. "A survey of augmented reality technologies, applications and limitations." *The International Journal of Virtual Reality* 9.2 (2010): 1–20.
11. Yuen, Steve Chi-Yin, Gallayanee Yaoyuneyong, and Erik Johnson. "Augmented reality: an overview and five directions for AR in education." *Journal of Educational Technology Development and Exchange (JETDE)* 4.1 (2011): 11.
12. Mewada, S., A. Saroliya, N. Chandramouli, T. Rajasanthosh Kumar, M. Lakshmi, S. Mary, and M. Jayakumar. "Smart diagnostic expert system for defect in forging process by using machine learning process." *Journal of Nanomaterials* 1 (2022): 2567194.
13. Alismail, Abdullah, et al. "Augmented reality glasses improve adherence to evidence-based intubation practice." *Advances in Medical Education and Practice* 2019 (2019): 279–286.
14. Starner, Thad, et al. "Augmented reality through wearable computing." *Presence Teleoperators and Virtual Environments* 6.4 (1997): 386–398.
15. Bottani, Eleonora, and Giuseppe Vignali. "Augmented reality technology in the manufacturing industry: a review of the last decade." *IISE Transactions* 51.3 (2019): 284–310.
16. Lovreglio, R., et al. "Digital technologies for fire evacuations." In Huang, X., Tam, W.C. (eds) *Intelligent Building Fire Safety and Smart Firefighting.* Springer Nature Switzerland, 2024. 439–454.
17. Rampolla, Joseph, and Greg Kipper. *Augmented Reality: An Emerging Technologies Guide to AR.* Elsevier, 2012.
18. Shirowzhan, Sara, Willie Tan, and Samad M. E. Sepasgozar. "Digital twin and CyberGIS for improving connectivity and measuring the impact of infrastructure construction planning in smart cities." *ISPRS International Journal of Geo-Information* 9.4 (2020): 240.
19. Lukosch, Stephan, et al. "Providing information on the spot: using augmented reality for situational awareness in the security domain." *Computer Supported Cooperative Work (CSCW)* 24 (2015): 613–664.
20. Agrawal, Ankit, and Jane Cleland-Huang. "RescueAR: augmented reality supported collaboration for UAV driven emergency response systems." *arXiv preprint arXiv:2110.00180* (2021).
21. Wang, Xiangyu, et al. "Augmented reality in built environment: classification and implications for future research." *Automation in Construction* 32 (2013): 1–13.
22. Shuhaiber, Jeffrey H. "Augmented reality in surgery." *Archives of Surgery* 139.2 (2004): 170–174.
23. Davis, Matthew Christopher, et al. "Virtual interactive presence in global surgical education: international collaboration through augmented reality." *World Neurosurgery* 86 (2016): 103–111.

24. Kohli, Varun, et al. "A review on virtual reality and augmented reality use-cases of brain computer interface based applications for smart cities." *Microprocessors and Microsystems* 88 (2022): 104392.
25. Siriwardhana, Yushan, et al. "A survey on mobile augmented reality with 5G mobile edge computing: architectures, applications, and technical aspects." *IEEE Communications Surveys & Tutorials* 23.2 (2021): 1160–1192.

CHAPTER 4

Assessing the Effectiveness of AR/VR-Based Fire Fighter Training

Santosh Reddy P, Supriya Sudhir, and Kalyani S Kumar

4.1 INTRODUCTION

Nowadays people spend 80%–90% of their lifetime inside massive, extravagant buildings. Navigating a building becomes more challenging with an increased number of occupants. Rescue teams are essential during an indoor disaster, such as a fire or gas leak, which may result in fatalities and significant property damage. The number of individuals preparing for an indoor emergency has increased. Engaging in several tasks within a complex environment might lead to fatigue among rescuers, hence complicating rescue efforts in such scenarios. Indoor disaster situations may provide obstacles like fire-related impediments, barriers, and unreliable communication [1]. Expeditious decision-making and execution are crucial for rescue teams to save lives; nevertheless, such efficacy may be hindered in this context. For example, delays in rescue operations may arise if teams encounter difficulties in sustaining communication with the command-and-control unit. The advancement of communication and protective equipment for rescue crews has led to much more complex rescue operations in recent years. However, there are few technologies available to assist rescue professionals in saving more lives during critical situations

DOI: 10.1201/9781003564904-4

[2]. Rescuers may need some time to ascertain a method for traversing a blocked interior space, such as one obstructed by fire or other impediments. Rescue teams may use mixed reality (MR) technology to simulate decision-making in various scenarios, hence reducing response times.

Virtual reality (VR) and augmented reality (AR) elements are combined in mixed reality. Interaction with virtual items in the physical realm and with tangible objects in a digital environment is feasible [3–5]. This enhances user immersion and effectively conveys the essential information by showcasing the significant attributes of digital objects. This principle was used in the construction of a hybrid indoor evacuation system. The majority of firefighting research concerning MR has been on training. This project included the development of a mixed-reality system to mimic indoor catastrophe rescue scenarios [6–14]. The technology simulates catastrophe situations, allowing the user to go to the location of the incident. It subsequently offers enhanced layout maps for travelling to designated locations to save people in diverse scenarios, before eventually exiting the catastrophe zone by multiple routes to conclude the lifesaving drill [15–19]. Researchers assessed the efficacy of the technology by analyzing the effectiveness of the rescue procedure concerning the "golden time," at which point smoke inhalation becomes fatal.

4.2 THE RELATED WORK

This unit provides an overview of disaster safety research based on MR and includes case studies of actual disasters.

4.2.1 Safety in Disasters

Disasters such as earthquakes and fires often result in widespread damage that exceeds the capacity of standard management and emergency response systems. These incidents often cause harm, destruction of property, and even fatalities; therefore they need an urgent and efficient reaction (particularly as they often occur without warning). Numerous research on safety in catastrophe circumstances has been conducted. The massive volume of information produced during catastrophes, or "big data," has prompted the creation of new safety tech in recent years to improve disaster responses. Blockchain technology, for instance, may be utilized to store and validate information to determine a catastrophe's cause. Using data from daily reports, Lee et al.'s research examined and categorized the characteristics of "cold wave" catastrophes. Munawar et al. used big data collection to assess the safety of infrastructure during natural catastrophes. Kaur and colleagues utilized IoT devices to collect big data for disaster prediction and evacuation.

Disaster management relies heavily on big data, including its collection, processing, and visualization. The goal of Alabdulaali et al. was to improve the readability of big data about disasters. The application of AI in disaster research has grown in tandem with the amount of study on big data as it pertains to disasters. Artificial intelligence was used by Ketmaneechairat and colleagues to transform audio recordings into text for automated catastrophe categorization. Using data collected from sensors and models trained using machine learning, Duggal et al. examined the frequency of disasters. In the event of a crisis, Zhao and colleagues used an AI model to determine the best escape route by analyzing user position data collected from sensors. In their study, Salmi et al. successfully detected earthquakes by combining geological vibration data using long short-term memory models based on convolutional neural networks. To forecast the occurrence of fires by analyzing smoke images, Majid and colleagues used models trained on convolutional neural networks. To identify whether an individual was wearing a disguise in camera-captured photos, Magherini et al. used a ResNet50 model of convolutional neural networks. In the aftermath of devastating fires, Ahn et al. utilized closed-circuit television (CCTV) video to identify blazes before they spread. To distinguish between "fire" and "normal" photos captured during wildfires, Khan et al. trained a deep learning model using video from actual fires. Using CCTV picture data, Huang et al. classified hazardous regions using the YOLOv3 algorithm. Yu et al. used a deep learning model to identify subterranean catastrophes. As a result, AI is crucial for catastrophe management and prevention. Knowing the state of the environment is critical in a crisis event.

A faster and more efficient reaction to disasters is possible with the help of data collected in real time from a variety of sensors made possible by the Internet of Things (IoT). Using IoT sensors, Anuradha and colleagues created a disaster safety monitoring method that records and tracks typical environmental factors like temperature, rainfall, and vibration to be ready for any calamities. By keeping an eye on electrical energy—a source of fires—Chhetri et al. used IoT sensors to identify possible catastrophes. Using underwater IoT sensors, Dai et al. developed a system for marine environment management. Nguyen et al. used IoT sensor technologies to find individuals who went missing after disasters. To improve the safety of rescue personnel during catastrophes, Brar et al. developed an IoT sensor–based disaster scenario decision-making system. The aforementioned research provides an overview of a few of the many safety and disaster management strategies that aid rescue professionals and victims by using early warning systems and real-time data.

4.2.2 Combined Virtual and Real

As an expansion of current VR technology, mixed reality exists on a continuum between the two extremes and incorporates both digital and physical items. Virtual reality and augmented reality are merging. Two types of objects may be found in a real-world setting: one is a virtual item, and the other is a digital version of a real-world thing. Mixed realism is seen in Figure 4.1.

Acampora et al. used a mixed-reality game to teach police personnel to identify offenders. With the use of mixed-reality apps, Gattullo et al. were able to enhance their lectures. Kabuye et al. created a surgical device that was quite realistic in its simulation of the procedure using mixed reality. Wu et al. utilized mixed reality to educate construction workers on the risks posed by various tools and materials used on the job site. During

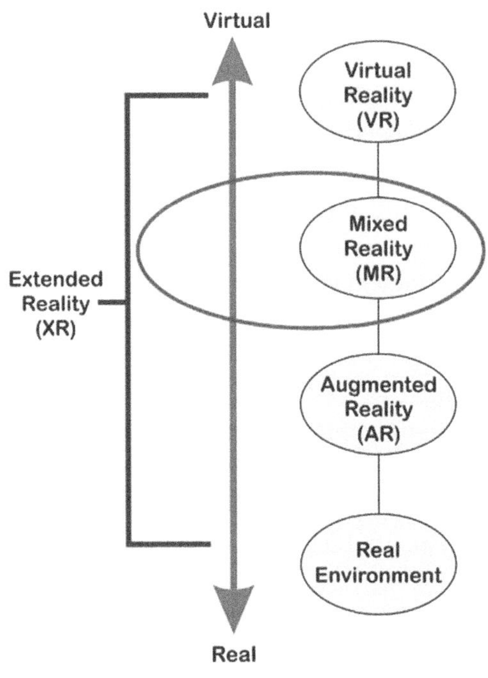

FIGURE 4.1 Mixed realism concepts.

human-robot cooperation, Choi et al. utilized virtual reality to maintain a safe distance between robots and people.

Applying mixed reality to real-time manufacturing operations, Mortzis et al. collaborated with supervisors and field workers in distant places. For remote robotic manipulation, Ulloa et al. used virtual reality. To improve training and rehabilitation, Franzo et al. used mixed reality to create a 3D virtual model that visualizes exercise posture in real time. Because there are such various uses for mixed reality, we thought it would help with disaster recovery.

4.3 METHODS AND MATERIALS

Indoor disaster reaction and teamwork using our MR system are detailed in the following, along with the scenario and design technique. Our system's MR hardware has an integrated mapping and localization sensor to gather spatial data. The MR device's internal algorithm is responsible for the mapping. The user must perform a simulation based on the mapped interior area to rescue persons who are trapped inside after an indoor catastrophe scenario. The user takes on the role of a fireman in the virtual world. To end the simulation, the user must get to the exit after the rescue mission. Two or more people may participate in the rescue missions depending on the scenarios. A schematic of the MR system that simulates an indoor catastrophe rescue is shown in Figure 4.2.

4.3.1 Hypothetical Situations

The user follows the navigation instructions to the room where the indoor catastrophe happened after activating the system, and then the status pane is triggered. Here the researcher will go over the many indoor disaster response situations that the MR system can mimic. After powering up the machine, the user follows the on-screen prompts to the exact location of the indoor catastrophe, and then the status window becomes active. In the event of a fire, virtual items are used as symbols. After the fire calamity, the user comes to the aid of the victims. Figure 4.3 shows a high-level perspective of a mock rescue mission.

Here are three possible outcomes that the MR system might mimic:

- Scenario 1 (S1): A simulated calamity happens in one area, and those who are stuck there are rescued by using the main staircase.
- Scenario 2 (S2): Two simulated disasters happen, and trapped people are rescued via the main staircase once more.

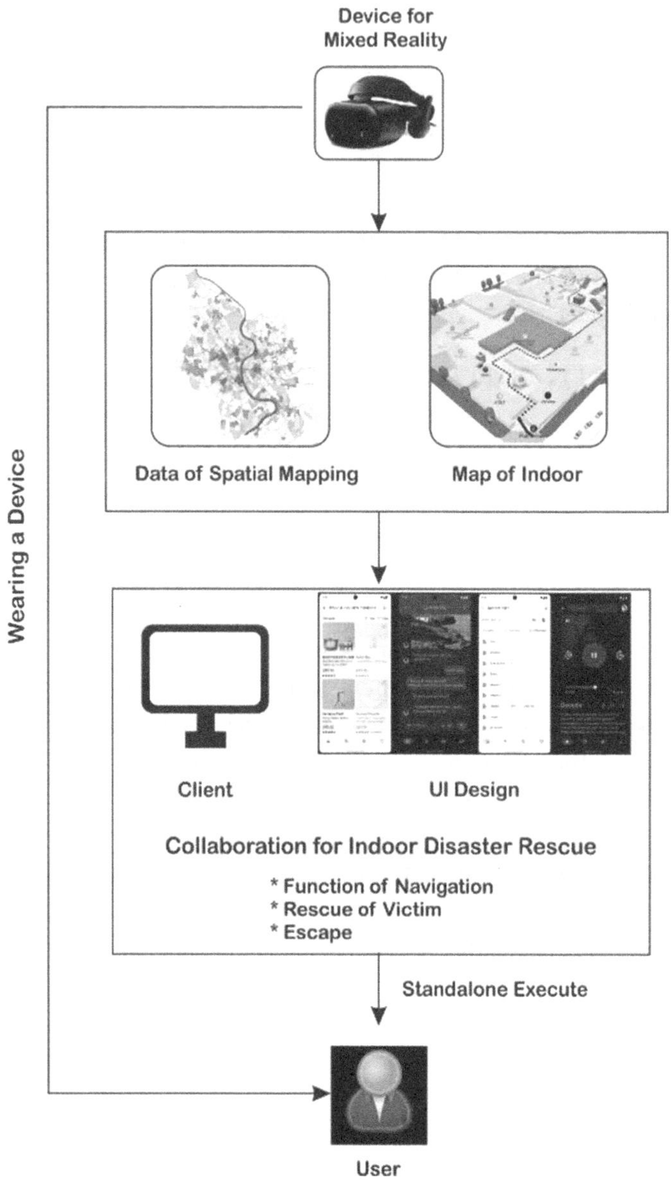

FIGURE 4.2 Schematic of the MR system that simulates an indoor catastrophe rescue.

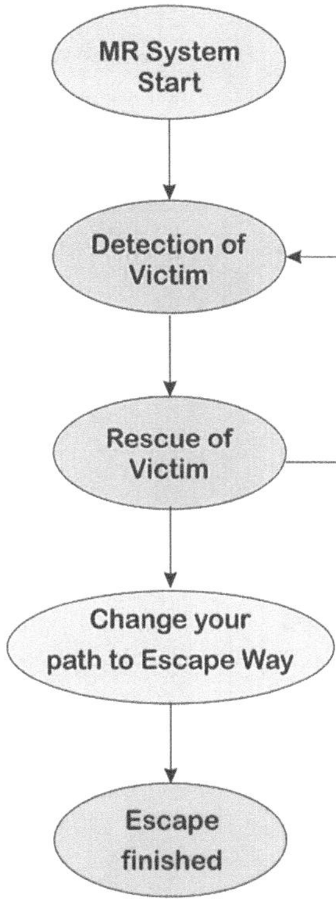

FIGURE 4.3 Perspective of a mock rescue mission.

- Scenario 3 (S3): In this scenario, a virtual calamity happens in a single area, and anybody who is trapped has to be rescued via the main staircase. The evacuation eventually takes place via a different exit, however, because of an unanticipated fire in a different hallway.

The algorithm makes use of a campus map. The "starting point" is the user's current position. You can see the big picture of the map and the scenarios in Figure 4.4.

4.3.2 Function of the System

The functioning of the system is detailed here. The user must first gather geographical data to determine their exact position. After that, the user's present location is shown while a simulated interior catastrophe scenario is created using this information. At startup, the system creates a map of the user's current position. After comparing the current location with the

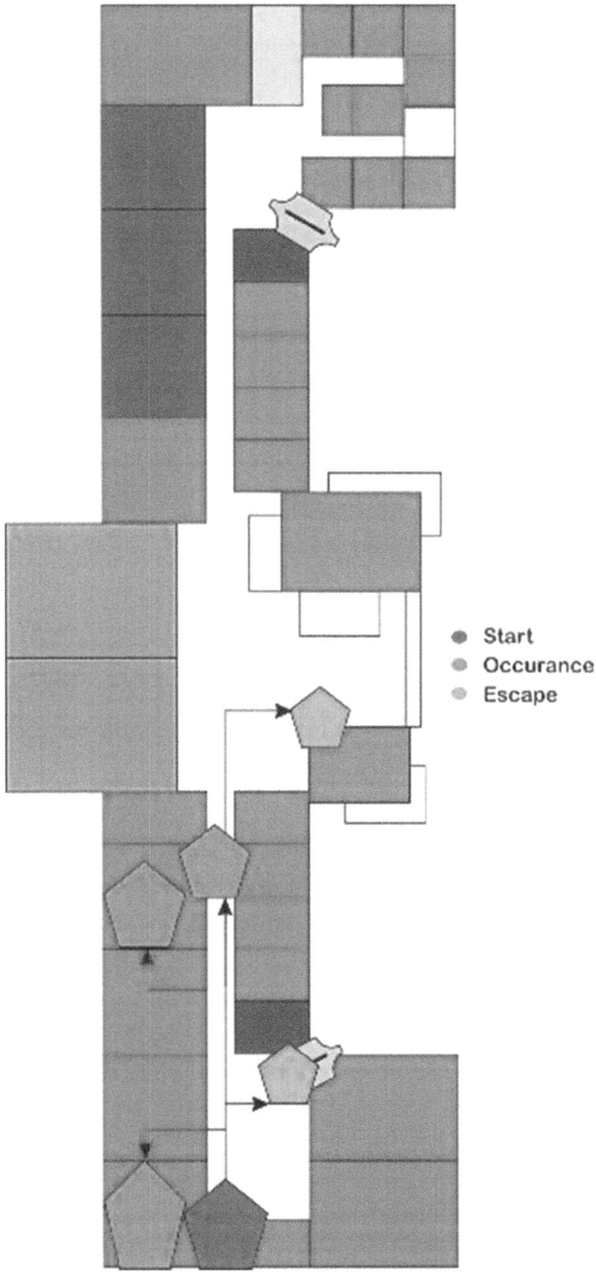

FIGURE 4.4 The big picture of the map and the scenarios.

stored mapping information, the operator's current position is shown on the interior map. A haphazard indoor catastrophe scenario is generated using the mapping data. Next, the user must go to the site of the indoor catastrophe. After that, they utilize the navigation feature, which displays distance and direction via arrows and a status pane. Upon reaching the site of the inside catastrophe, the user is tasked with finding and rescuing any survivors. After everyone has been saved, the user may go to the main staircase to exit. Figure 4.5 shows the MR system's operating sequence.

4.3.3 System Designing

Here you may find the Unity stages that were used to develop the MR system. The left-handed position system is used for object movement and rotation in Unity. The system automatically adds a user-position indicator to the indoors map as it starts up. The camera is then rotated 90 degrees along the *X*-axis and 180 degrees along the *Y*-axis, while the *Z*-axis remains fixed, to reveal the indoor map and user position indicator from the front. This design allows you to manage movement by rotating the map along the *X*-axis and to see the user's position icon (depending on the *X*-axis value) by rotating it along the *Z*-axis, without effecting the *Y*-axis rotation. One component of the system's design is a mechanism for fine-tuning the user's icon position on the static indoor map display. After adding the starting point to the *X* and *Z* coordinate values, dividing by 5, and applying the position correction values, the desired result is obtained. Because the hardware's coordinates vary from the program's, calibration is required. In Unity's coordinate system, five pixels represent the movement of the "1.0 coordinates values" as they move across the screen. The indoor map, with the method's user position symbol shown (Figure 4.6), is presented.

The user may view their present direction, the next direction, the distance, and the time it will take to go to the next destination after the system has begun and the status window has been opened. Because updating the status information is necessary for applying the computed values to the status display, Unity's thread processing functionality is essential. A request is sent to the main thread by the socket thread because it lacks access to the status window. The next step is to establish a queue and make it available to the main thread. When data is queued, the socket thread moves it along. When new information becomes available that would necessitate updating the status window's presented information, the main thread of Unity checks the queue size and makes the necessary

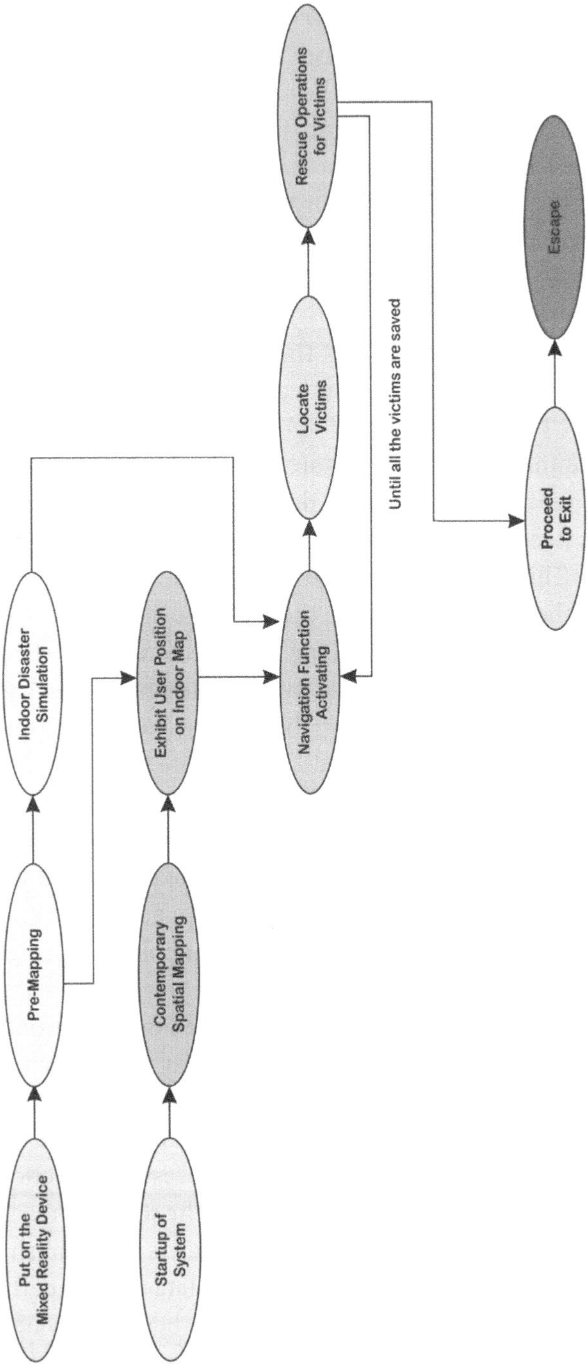

FIGURE 4.5 MR system's operating sequence.

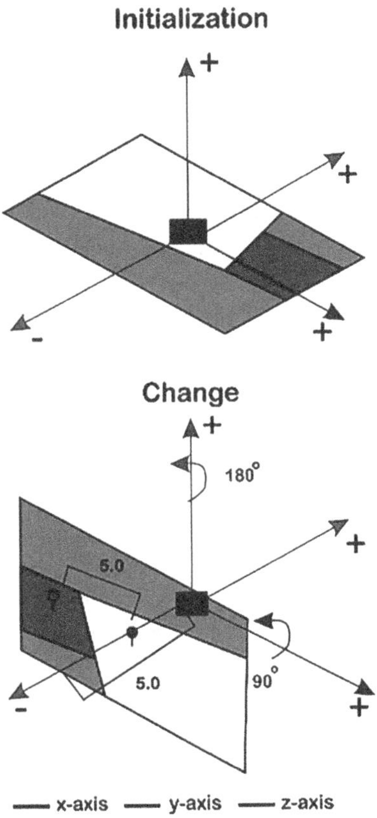

FIGURE 4.6 Indoor map with the system's user position icon.

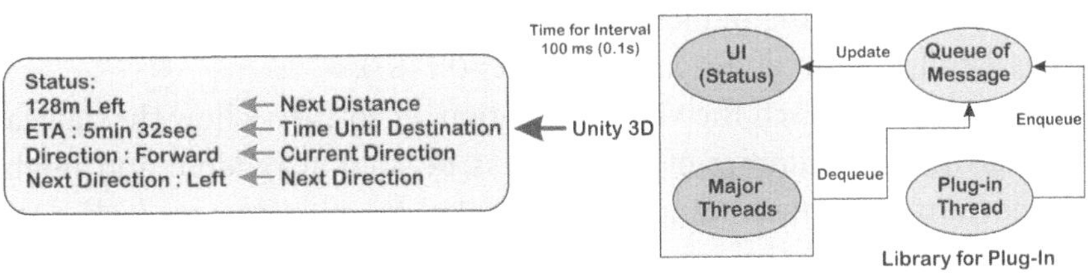

FIGURE 4.7 Procedures shown in the status pane.

modifications. The procedures shown in the status pane are illustrated in Figure 4.7.

Upon activation of the MR system, a virtual interior catastrophe scenario is produced at random, complete with a virtual victim. Upon completion of the rescue, an exit point is constructed. The user is intended to have the navigation function presented to them as an arrow. The navigation arrow changes direction according to the angle of the axis where the victim is positioned, guiding the user to their location. After applying a correction value of 0.5, the arrow remains in its original position pointing at the victim; it only rotates from this position to help with interpretation. When a victim is rescued, an escape point is established. The navigation arrow changes direction according to the angle of the escape path. The simulation is set up such that the y-axis value is <0 to represent an escape, as exits often contain numerous steps. You can see the navigation feature in Figure 4.8.

The MR system, as mentioned before, plays out scenarios where victims must be rescued in the event of a tragedy. Data about previously mapped locations is saved in the device's memory. When turned on, the system asynchronously creates simulated disaster locations and victims at random. Each victim has a corresponding button that, when pressed, deactivates the item representing them, allowing for their rescue.

4.3.4 Client for System

At launch, the system initializes the user's location so it can learn more about the system client. You can see the status window, the user's position indicator, and the directional arrow on the indoor map. These processes are running in the background when the computer boots up. On the indoor map, the user's location is displayed by the number 1. Number 2 is the navigation tool that takes the client to the scene of the catastrophe. Number 3 represents the function that indicates the distances and the anticipated time to escape. Number 4 represents the sites of the simulated disasters. Finally, the number 5 represents the victim. Section 4.3.1 provides a full account of the circumstances (S1–S3).

The user will reach the victim's location when they follow the navigation arrow. The number of casualties is decided at random and might range from one to four. In situations S1–S3, the victim is rescued when the user reaches the victim's position and hits the button on the victim's bottom. When all victims have been rescued, the navigational aids leading to the exit will be turned on.

Following the navigational instructions, the player must go towards the exit after saving a victim. Most exits in a normal building are located on the upper floors. According to the scenario in Section 4.3.2, the system may be shut off and the escape can be completed by descending from the fourth to the third level. This is in line with S1 and S2 situations and the steps used to rescue the victim and make their way to the exit.

An unforeseen fire breaks out in the centre corridor as the rescuers rush for the exit, saving the victim in the process. Here, the navigation arrow points away from the present exit and towards an alternate exit.

4.4 RESULTS

This section details the assessment of the system's performance and its surroundings. The aforementioned Unity is capable of handling VR/AR systems, and it is also used by the planned MR system.

When it comes to saving lives, time is of the essence. More than 60% of fire fatalities are attributable to smoke and gas inhalation, making the first five minutes of a fire the most crucial for rescuing survivors. Thus, rescuing people within 5 minutes is the objective of the exercises. Based on this time constraint, this system included ten experimenters (eight male and two female). Out of these, three had prior experience with MR settings (VR or AR) and seven had no such background. Although many complicated factors are involved in rescue efforts in real-world catastrophe scenarios, escue operations may be made easier in simulated catastrophe scenarios. For the rescue scenarios, the golden time was therefore shortened from 5 minutes to 2 minutes. To proceed, one must do things like put out a fire or clear the path. If this had been taken into account when designing the system, the experiment should have been scheduled to take place during prime time. However, because it was intended to ensure that people could be saved by touch alone, it was estimated that it would take one minute and thirty seconds to put out the fire or remove the obstruction, so the timer was set for two minutes. There was a total of three experiments overseen by each experimenter for each scenario. Participants' ability to quickly rescue the victim or victims and flee served as a measure of the MR method's effectiveness. Figure 4.8 displays the scenario indices. Scenarios S1–S3 cover managing unexpected occurrences, accuracy, and speed in that sequence.

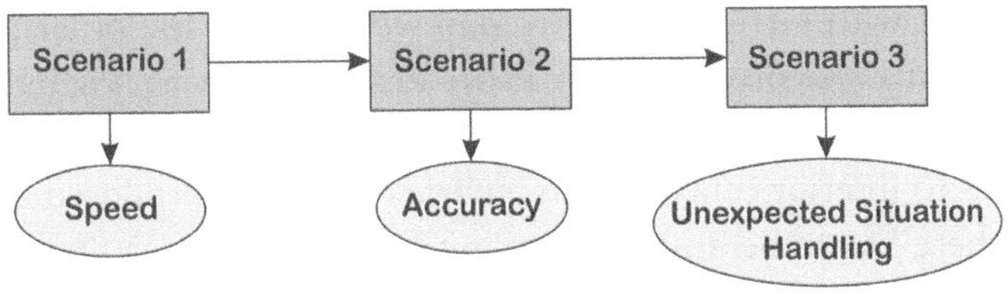

FIGURE 4.8 Scenario indices.

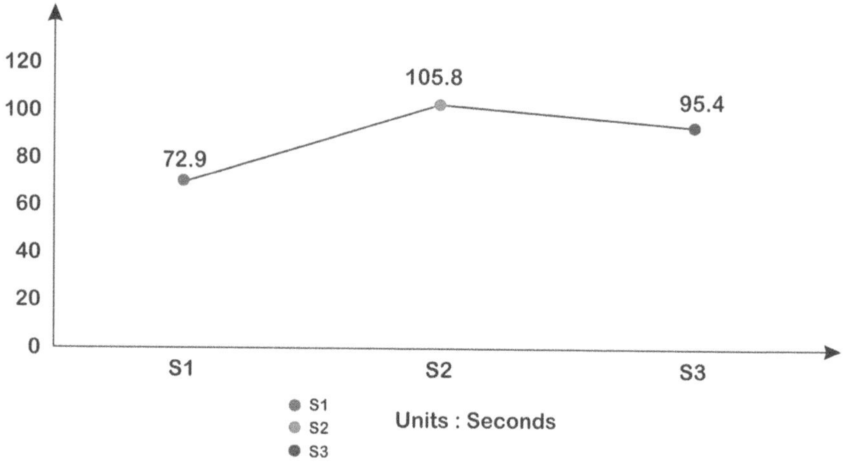

FIGURE 4.9 Average amount of time needed to leave in each case.

Figure 4.9 illustrates the general times it takes to get away in all three situations. The last people to finish the project were asked to give feedback that would help guide future study that aims to improve the method.

In S1, the golden time for rescue and escape was significantly reduced, showing that the system's navigational guidance can speedily rescue victims and then allow the rescuer to flee to safety. The golden time was similarly reduced in S2 and S3. Consequently, the amount of time needed to re-explore to escape from an unforeseen circumstance was decreased. The system's efficacy was shown, on average, by the golden time reduction. Rescue efforts in confined spaces were therefore made easier by the MR system.

To enhance the MR system, it is crucial to prioritize the input from participants and make it compatible with numerous devices. While testing the system, a second person stood at the user's side and manually interacted with the virtual items. We are working on making the system more compatible with MR devices so that it may be utilized with more of them. Reducing spatial location inaccuracy, enhancing rescue operations, and dealing with virtual object overlap were among the other proposed enhancements. Incorporating real-life rescue tools as virtual objects allows for more accurate simulations, which is essential for training responses to interior catastrophe scenarios using the proposed approach. Lastly, there has to be an improvement in the cumulative inaccuracy of indoor spatial locations. Sensors included in the system enable spatial navigation and the projection of virtual things into physical space. Nevertheless, position error—that is, differences between the virtual object's location and real-world space coordinates—accumulates with continued system usage. Consequently, there is a demand for strategies and approaches that may decrease this mistake.

4.5 CONCLUSION

The goal of MR-based technology is to facilitate a safe, efficient, and quick rescue operation in the event of an indoor accident. To test how well the system worked, crisis scenarios were simulated where rescuers had just two minutes to complete their missions. Results showed that participants improved their speed by 39.3%, their accuracy by 11.9%, and their ability to respond to unexpected events by 20.6% in S1–S3, for a total increase of 23.9%. The suggested system is shown to be efficient by these outcomes. The participants also offered suggestions for enhancements, such as making the system compatible with more devices. It is also important to handle issues like object overlap and cumulative spatial mapping mistakes. To encourage a quicker reaction time to disasters and guarantee the safety of rescuers and firemen, the suggested MR system mimics rescue operations.

REFERENCES

1. Koutitas, George, Scott Smith, and Grayson Lawrence. "Performance evaluation of AR/VR training technologies for EMS first responders." *Virtual Reality* 25.1 (2021): 83–94.
2. Chen, Haosen, et al. "Development of BIM, IoT and AR/VR technologies for fire safety and upskilling." *Automation in Construction* 125 (2021): 103631.
3. Gong, Peizhen, et al. "Applications and effectiveness of augmented reality in safety training: a systematic literature review and meta-analysis." *Safety Science* 178 (2024): 106624.
4. Rathore, P. S., Ahuja, S., Burri, S. R., Khunteta, A., Baliyan, A., & Kumar, A. (2024). *Deep learning techniques for automation and industrial applications.* John Wiley & Sons, Inc.; Scrivener Publishing LLC.
5. Kang, Hosan, et al. "Integrated augmented and virtual reality technologies for realistic fire drill training." *IEEE Computer Graphics and Applications* 44, 2 (2023): 89–99.
6. Vukelic, Goran, et al. "Application of VR technology for maritime firefighting and evacuation training—a review." *Journal of Marine Science and Engineering* 11.9 (2023): 1732.
7. Mewada, Shivlal, Anil Saroliya, N. Chandramouli, T. Rajasanthosh Kumar, M. Lakshmi, S. Suma Christal Mary, and Mani Jayakumar. "Research article smart diagnostic expert system for defect in forging process by using machine learning process." *System (In Section 4)* 19 (2022): 21.
8. Yang, Li, et al. "Train and equip firefighters with cognitive virtual and augmented reality." *2018 IEEE 4th International Conference on Collaboration and Internet Computing (CIC)*. IEEE, 2018.

9. Paes, Daniel, Zhenan Feng, Susan Mander, Selim Datoussaid, Thierry Descamps, Anass Rahouti, and Ruggiero Lovreglio. "Video see-through augmented reality fire safety training: A comparison with virtual reality and video training." *Safety Science* 184 (2025): 106714.
10. Berthiaume, Maxine, et al. "Evaluation of a virtual reality training tool for firefighters responding to transportation incidents with dangerous goods." *Education and Information Technologies* 29 (2024): 1–39.
11. BramahHazela, J. Hymavathi, T. Rajasanthosh Kumar, S. Kavitha, D. Deepa, Sachin Lalar, and Prabakaran Karunakaran. "Machine Learning: Supervised Algorithms to Determine the Defect in High-Precision Foundry Operation." *Journal of Nanomaterials* 2022 (1) (2022): 1732441.
12. Koutitas, George, Scott Smith, Grayson Lawrence, and Keith Noble. "Smart responders for smart cities: A VR/AR training approach for next generation first responders." In *Smart Cities in Application: Healthcare, Policy, and Innovation*, pp. 49–66. Cham: Springer International Publishing, 2019.
13. Liu, Xiao-Wei, et al. "Research on training effectiveness of professional maintenance personnel based on virtual reality and augmented reality technology." *Sustainability* 14.21 (2022): 14351.
14. Kim, Kyungki, et al. "Using immersive augmented reality to assess the effectiveness of construction safety training." *Journal of Construction Engineering and Project Management* 9.4 (2019): 16–33.
15. Khanal, Shishir, et al. "Virtual and augmented reality in the disaster management technology: a literature review of the past 11 years." *Frontiers in Virtual Reality* 3 (2022): 843195.
16. Kapalo, Katelynn A., Patricia Bockelman, and Joseph J. LaViola Jr. ""Sizing Up" Emerging Technology for Firefighting: Augmented Reality for Incident Assessment." *Proceedings of the Human Factors and Ergonomics Society Annual Meeting* 62.1 (2018): 1464–1468.
17. del Carmen Cardós-Alonso, María, et al. "Extended reality training for mass casualty incidents: a systematic review on effectiveness and experience of medical first responders." *International Journal of Emergency Medicine* 17.1 (2024): 99.
18. Redford, Amy Caryn. *Perceptions of the use of augmented and virtual reality supporting emergency response education and training*. Dissertation. Capella University, 2021.
19. Xie, Biao, et al. "A review on virtual reality skill training applications." *Frontiers in Virtual Reality* 2 (2021): 645153.

CHAPTER 5

Simulation-Based Training with Augmented Reality for Paramedics

Charanjeet Singh, Hariballav Mahapatra, Malini R, Kavitha G L, and Kiran Sree Pokkuluri

5.1 INTRODUCTION

A disaster is an unexpected event that has the potential to kill people and destroy a lot of property [1–3]. The sort of calamity and the conditions in which individuals find themselves determine how quickly these situations might deteriorate [4]. No amount of preparation will ever fully protect people from witnessing or suffering the death of loved ones in such tragedies [3, 5, 6].

Despite advances in science and technology, such as weather forecasting methods, the harm that natural catastrophes bring to resources and human life cannot be stopped [7–9]. Nature has repeatedly shown itself to be significantly stronger than humans [10]. In certain cases, such as earthquakes and tsunamis, there is only a short period to prepare for the disaster [11–15]. The success of adaptive as well as coping techniques can be measured by whether the necessary skills, knowledge, and resources are prepared ahead of time and can be used quickly when needed [16, 17]. So, it is evident that several building, community, and personal safety measures can significantly mitigate the negative consequences of natural catastrophes [18–21].

Augmented and virtual reality (AR/VR) are among the most rapidly expanding technological fields in the world [22]. Most notably, the gaming

DOI: 10.1201/9781003564904-5

and entertainment industries make heavy use of AR/VR. Many other industries make heavy use of AR/VR as well, including healthcare, education, e-commerce, the automobile industry, the military, and real estate [23]. Emergency management programs do not often take advantage of these technologies [24]. Some examples of augmented reality applications include Google Maps, gaming (e.g., Pikmin Bloom), military defence (e.g., AR goggles), and retail (e.g., World Market).

The objective is to create disaster preparation software that uses augmented reality to provide users with a better experience of a catastrophic event, such as a fire. As a result, users will be exposed to a variety of realistic scenarios in this program, getting ready for any possible variables like fear, worry, and so on.

5.2 INDIA'S AR AND VR TRENDS

- Security: The Indian army (Tamil Nadu) uses Imaginate's VR platform, ShootAR.
- LiveVR in healthcare: Helping with complicated operations.
- Meraki for enjoyment.
- Properties such as Makaan, the website Housing.com, etc.
- Byjus' Institute.
- Automobiles: MG Motor Company and Avataar's partnership.
- Digital commerce: StyleDotMe.

5.3 OBJECTIVES

- Design an augmented reality app.
- Make icons for the app's menu.
- Conduct photo recognition scans by employing smart card technology.
- Integrate interactive virtual buttons to enhance UI.

- Develop the prototype with a focus on home fire threats.
- Arrange three-dimensional items on the card's front side.
- Fill up the card's back side with pertinent information.

5.4 SURVEY OF LITERATURE

Virtual and augmented worlds have been used, with their pros and cons and their potential in many areas, such as crisis planning. Studies are still being done on these topics.

The chapter [3] asserts that disaster preparation is crucial to lowering the number of fatalities in the event of a catastrophe. According to the report, India loses over a billion dollars annually as a result of calamities. This figure is an essential warning that money has to be spent on innovative techniques to make people more resilient in these circumstances.

Augmented reality and virtual reality have been used a lot in the main areas of protective system architecture, human behaviour research, and emergency safety training. The area for studying human behaviour had almost 27 designs, and all of them were based on VR. Now, there are currently almost 19 plans for emergency safety training, with 13 being VR-based and 8 being AR-based.

In order to better train rescue teams, the researchers have detailed the usage of augmented reality. The user may pinpoint their exact position by seeing a virtual panorama. Through the app's user interface, the trainer may manage all of the processes. Although the concept was successful, more thorough research and evaluation were required.

Many different kinds of AR systems are described in the work. The three primary kinds of augmented reality identified in this research are location-based augmentation, dynamic augmentation, and complex augmentation. Ideas are discussed for how to use virtual reality tools to help people who have been affected by earthquakes at work. Some of the gear that has been used is a stand, a GPS device, video cameras, and an Inertial Measurement Device. A real-life picture is mixed with a computer-generated picture made by 3D graphics software to make the combination. The video stream from the camera is only used as the foundation of the scene shown in the 3D graphics application if the camera choice is chosen. For smaller problems, the plan worked properly.

5.5 STATISTICS ON PROTOTYPE

5.5.1 Real-Life Example

Researchers have created an application that makes use of picture recognition–based augmented reality, also known as marker-based AR. The smart cards whose sides serve as target pictures for the program to scan to identify these photos in real time are developed. By creating a realistic-looking fire that emerges upon detecting a ground plane, we have also integrated markerless augmented reality. Figure 5.1 shows the overview of the smart card.

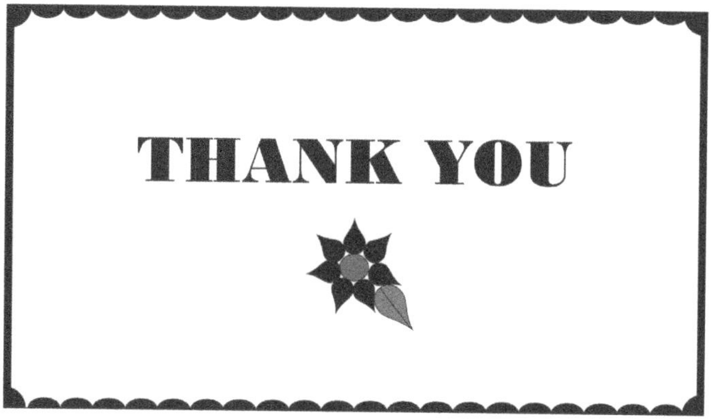

A. Backside 1

B. Backside 2

FIGURE 5.1 Overview of smart cards. (A) Backside 1, and (B) backside 2.

5.5.1.1 Technology

The following are prerequisites for creating an AR application:

- **System for Creating 3D Models in Real Time**:
  - To create 3D models and visuals, the researcher employed Blender, which was then imported into the Unity program.
  - The 3D project is created using Unity 3D and includes virtual objects (imported from Blender) and target pictures (which must be scanned).
- **Application Development Kit**:
  - Due to the compatibility with Unity 3D and its ability to install an augmented reality application based on markers on Android smartphones, the Vuforia engine is now being utilized for this purpose.
  - While working on the augmented reality project in Unity, we generated a license key using the Vuforia engine.
  - Checking the augmentable scores of our target photos was likewise done using Vuforia's online database.
- **Application-Deployment Device**:
  - The application is currently only available on Android smartphones.

5.5.1.2 Design of Algorithm

Figure 5.2 describes the step-by-step process of working on the smart cards in the proposed techniques.

5.5.1.3 Level of Technological Availability

Many different types of calamities could potentially be better prepared for with the use of AR and VR technology. Because of this, the project's scope is quite flexible. Domestic fire hazards are the current focus of the developed software. But there are a lot of different kinds of fire dangers and dangerous circumstances that might be included.

Therefore, the present degree of technological preparedness is a five on a scale ranging from one to nine. Figure 5.3 shows the AR with a marker while Figure 5.4 depicts the AR with the absence of a marker.

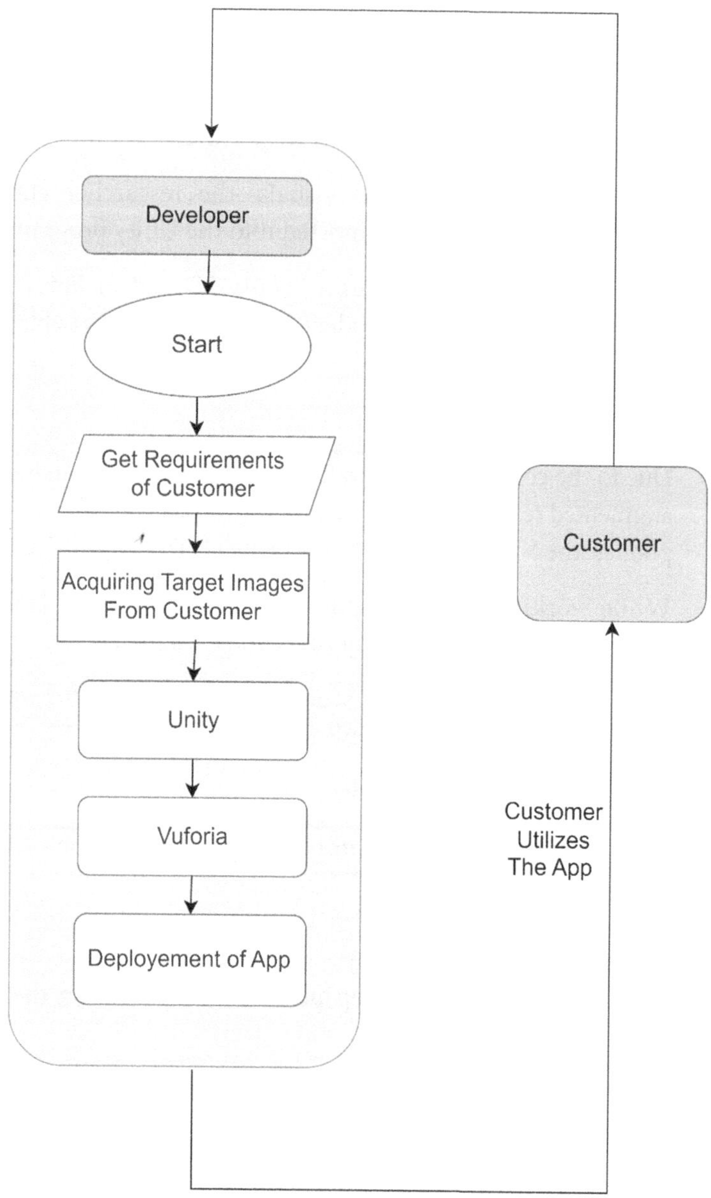

FIGURE 5.2 Flowchart for algorithm.

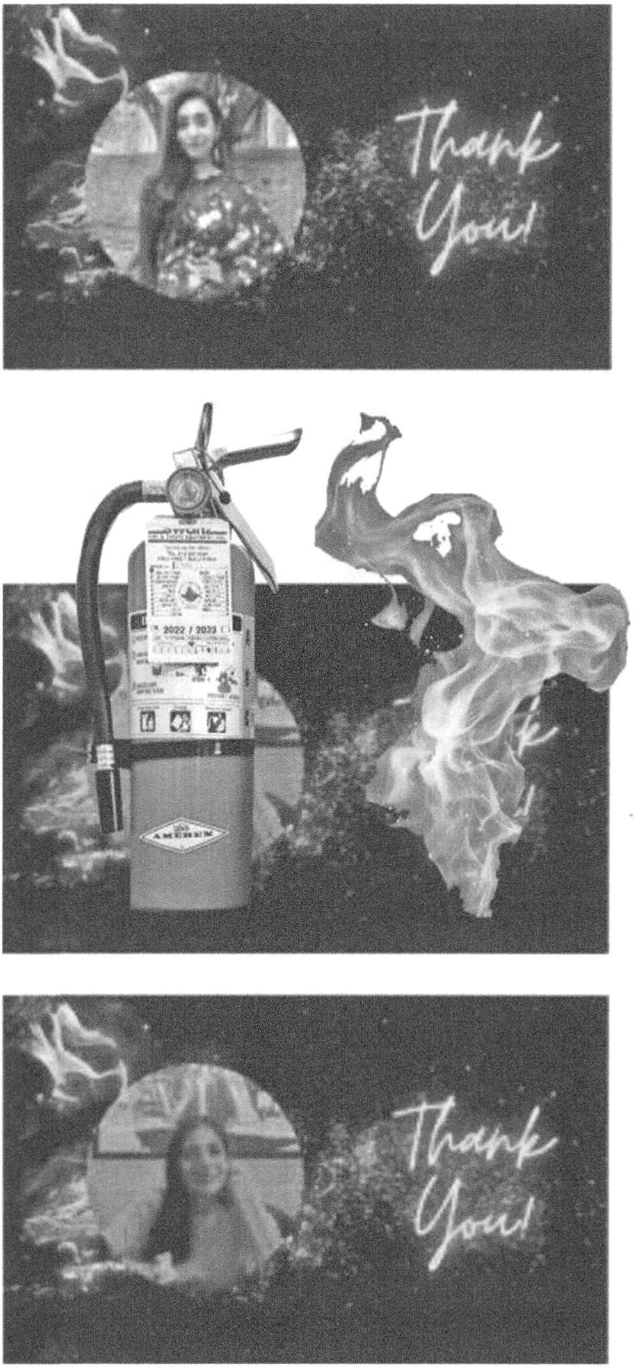

FIGURE 5.3 AR with marker.

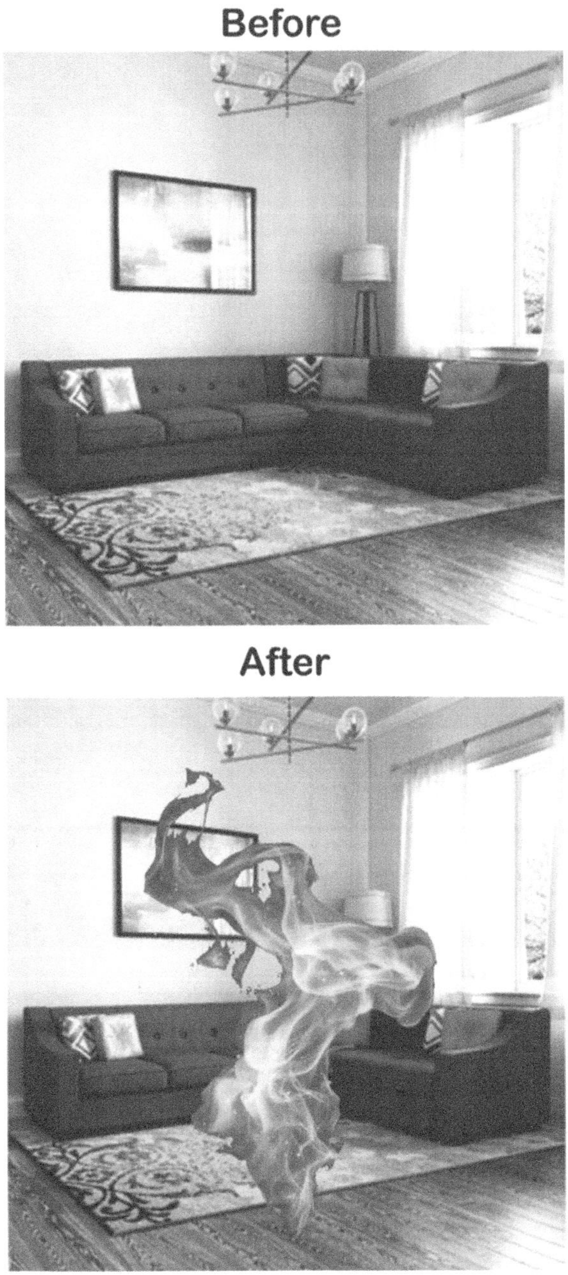

FIGURE 5.4 AR with no marker.

5.6 MERITS AND DEMERITS

5.6.1 Merits

A revolutionary new technology, AR allows users to seamlessly integrate the digital and physical worlds, resulting in dynamic, interactive settings that may be explored in novel ways. AR creates a whole new realm of interaction by superimposing digitally created visuals, audio, and other sensory data onto a user's actual surroundings. Users are not just passively viewing digital information; they can likewise interact with virtual elements, reveal hidden aspects of the real world, and perform actions that were previously impossible.

Bringing obscured objects into the consumer's view is a key function of augmented reality. One use of improved application of AR is to simulate the feeling of being in a burning building without putting the individual in danger. Similarly, virtual reality allows the user to visualize and interact with objects that are otherwise difficult or impossible to see, such as distant planets or microscopic organisms. These technologies offer users immediate access powerful instructional and experiential opportunities that were previously out of reach. A more detailed explanation of how AR benefits students and instructors is provided here:

1. Develops novel interactive encounters
2. Captures the hidden
3. Encourages active participation in education
4. Boosts academic possibilities
5. Promotes analytical reasoning and issue solving
6. Enhances understanding of concepts
7. Encourages originality and progress
8. Adjusts the classroom setting
9. Enhances memorization and comprehension
10. Makes higher education more available

In conclusion, AR offers tremendous potential to fill in knowledge gaps, foster creativity, and improve education. AR revolutionizes the way families interact with information and helps them better grasp complex concepts by creating meaningful and immersive experiences that integrate the virtual and real worlds. AR has the ability to bring about a paradigm shift in education by reinforcing conceptual understanding and critical thinking, creativity, and collaboration.

5.6.2 Demerits

1. Complexity of AR technology
2. A crash course on real and virtual components
3. Mobile augmented reality's dependability
4. Obstacles faced by interface designers
5. Issues with usability for target audiences
6. User anticipation versus actual experience
7. Ensuring device compatibility and support
8. Threats to transparency and safety
9. Constraints on technology
10. Updates and maintenance

In conclusion, improved reality has plenty of promise, but it still has a lot of questions with usability and common sense. Complexity, conflicting perceptions of real and virtual components, unstable tracking performance, unintuitive user interfaces, and concerns about accessibility are a few of the issues that can hinder the adoption and effective use of augmented reality. To overcome these obstacles, AR developers should focus on making interfaces foolproof, ensuring device compatibility across platforms, giving consumers clear directions, and addressing privacy and security concerns.

5.7 RESTRICTIONS

During the development of mobile augmented reality experiences, both users and developers encounter a range of challenges, including technological and non-technical issues.

Technical:

- Due to low light and poor camera quality, objects and images seem hazy and warped, and their colours begin to fade.

- Mobile augmented reality applications are notoriously power hogs as they need to activate the camera.

Non-technological:

- Despite the visually appealing nature of mobile AR, users may find it annoying to always have their phone nearby.

5.8 EFFECTS OF THE RESEARCH

Scientific studies have shown that AR considerably increases users' ability to learn when compared to more traditional methods. This is especially evident in fields where AR provides a more engaging, immersive, and practical learning experience, such as fire safety and emergency preparedness. Augmented reality apps may simulate real emergency scenarios, making fire security exercises more engaging and impactful than conventional methods that rely on paper information materials or classroom lectures.

1. Improve education and participation
2. Live-action crisis model
3. Training that is both accessible and convenient
4. Save money without sacrificing training
5. Ease of use and adaptability
6. Immediate criticism and assessment
7. Switch out paper-pen approaches
8. Possibilities for the future and general acceptance

As a conclusion, AR fire safety instruction is a better, more accessible, and cheaper option than the traditional approach. Augmented reality is a great tool for crisis response training since it can simulate real-life scenarios and provide users with quick feedback. As augmented reality becomes more widely used as an emergency preparedness tool, a significant shift is expected in how individuals are trained to respond to fires and other disasters.

5.9 CONCLUSION

The term "disaster preparedness" describes measures approved to reduce the impact of and prevent natural disasters. Among the various components of preparedness, training represents one of the most crucial. People in the community may be trained to help reduce the number of catastrophe victims and save lives. Virtual reality and augmented reality are two emerging technologies that may offer innovative ways to prepare individuals for hazardous situations. To enhance fire safety awareness, researchers developed a mobile augmented reality app. In the same way, AR and VR can be used to train people for many types of disaster scenarios.

REFERENCES

1. Aukstakalnis, S. *Practical Augmented Reality: A Guide to the Technologies, Applications, and Human Factors for AR and VR*. Addison-Wesley, 2016.
2. Sibilio, Maurizio, et al. "MetaWelt: Embodied in Which Body? Simplex Didactics to Live the Web 3.0." *International Conference on Human-Computer Interaction*. Cham: Springer Nature Switzerland, 2023.
3. Heim, Michael R. "Virtual reality wave 3." In J. Gackenbach & J. Bown (eds) *Boundaries of Self and Reality Online*. Academic Press, 2017. 261–277.
4. Crea, Teresa. *Integrating practice-based and neuroscientific perspectives on the impact of digital technology on contemporary narrative dramaturgy, investigated through live simulation exercises*. Dissertation. 2013.
5. Furia, Carlo A., et al. *Modelling Time in Computing*. Springer Science & Business Media, 2012.
6. Hymavathi, J., T. Rajasanthosh Kumar, S. Kavitha, D. Deepa, S. Lalar, and P. Karunakaran. "Machine learning: supervised algorithms to determine the defect in high-precision foundry operation." *Journal of Nanomaterials* 2022 (2022): 1–9.
7. Rathore, P. S., S. Ahuja, S. R. Burri, A. Khunteta, A. Baliyan, & A. Kumar (2024a). *Deep learning techniques for automation and industrial applications*. John Wiley & Sons, Inc.; Scrivener Publishing LLC.
8. Gualeni, Stefano. "Augmented ontologies: the question concerning digital technology and projectual humanism." (2014). https://repub.eur.nl/pub/51147/
9. De Groot, Jean. *Aristotle's Empiricism*. Parmenides Publishing, 2014.
10. Qvortrup, Lars. "Cyberspace as a representation of space experience: in defence of a phenomenological approach." In L. Qvortrup, J.F. Jensen, E. Kjems, N. Lehmann, and C. Madsen (eds) *Virtual space: Spatiality in virtual inhabited 3D worlds*. Springer, 2002. 5–24.
11. Dhotre, V.K. Anna, H.M., P.K. Pathak, A. Shrivastava, and T. Rajasanthosh Kumar. "Big data analytics using MapReduce for education system." *Linguistica Antverpiensia* 1 (2021): 3130–3138.
12. Wen, C.L. "Telemedicine, ehealth and remote care systems." In Heimar de Fátima Marin, Marco Antonio Gutierrez, Daniel Sigulem, Eduardo Massad, and Roberto J. Rodrigues (eds) *Global Health Informatics*. Academic Press, 2017. 168–194.

13. Ogleby, Cliff L. "From rubble to virtual reality: photogrammetry and the virtual world of ancient AYUTTHAYA, Thailand." *The Photogrammetric Record* 16.94 (1999): 651–670.
14. Tobias, Michael Charles, and Jane Gray Morrison "Metaphorical realities." In Michael Charles Tobias, Jane Gray Morrison *On the Nature of Ecological Paradox*. Springer International Publishing, 2021. 667–677.
15. Santaniello, Domenico. "Machine learning techniques and models for situation awareness of IoT based complex systems." (2022). http://elea.unisa.it/handle/10556/7239
16. Milani, Raffaele. *Dawn of a New Feeling: The Neocontemplative Condition*. McGill-Queen's Press-MQUP, 2022.
17. Cox, Hans Frederick. *Line-Storm: An Interactive Augmented Stylus and Writing Pad for Creative Human Performance*. University of Colorado Colorado Springs, 2018.
18. Gualeni, Stefano. *Virtual Worlds as Philosophical Tools: How to Philosophize with a Digital Hammer*. Springer, 2015.
19. Donlan, Joseph E. *Ordaining Reality: How Physics and Metaphysics Shape Your Future*. Universal-Publishers, 2021.
20. Devine, Kit. *Testing times: virtual heritage, 'time travel' and the user experience of museum visitors: a case study of an enriched time-based virtual heritage world*. Dissertation. The Australian National University (Australia), 2016.
21. Qvortrup, Lars. "Cyberspace as Representation of." In Lars Qvortrup, Jens F. Jensen, Erik Kjems, Niels Lehmann, Claus Madsen (eds) *Virtual Space: Spatiality in Virtual Inhabited 3D Worlds*. Springer, 2002. 1.
22. Di Tore, Pio Alfredo, ed. *A Simplex Approach to Learning, Cognition, and Spatial Navigation: Emerging Research and Opportunities: Emerging Research and Opportunities*. IGI Global, 2017.
23. Joy, Jimmy. *The Mind's Eye: The Evolution of the Athlete's Skills and Consciousness*. Lulu.Com, 2009. https://www.google.co.in/books/edition/The_Mind_s_Eye_The_Evolution_of_the_Athl/wPxyAgAAQBAJ?hl=en&gbpv=0
24. Bevolo, Marco, and Filiberto Amati. "The future of business events in the "phygital" age: development of a generative tool: a qualitative research project combining Design Research and foresight principles to co-design and develop a future matrix for potential implementation by business event designers and managers." *World Leisure Journal* 66.1 (2024): 92–115.

CHAPTER 6

Cost-Benefit Analysis of AR/VR Integration in Emergency Response

Lakshminarayana Reddy Kothapalli Sondinti, Venkata Krishna Azith Teja Ganti, Majjari Venkata Kesava Kumar, Vishwanadham Mandala, and R. Senthamil Selvan

6.1 INTRODUCTION

Pumping equipment has several maintenance guidelines. First, several guidelines centre on safety precautions [1]. Monitoring the pumping equipment's status allows for diagnostics and maintenance to be carried out when required. The concept of scheduled maintenance comes next. Based on their findings, engineers can foretell when and what kind of technical and service operations will be required to keep the pump running well. Third, there are the rules that govern reactive measures, which include fixing broken or malfunctioning equipment after the fact [2]. A backup plan for pump maintenance is to have some spare parts on hand and swap them out as needed. The running corporation is hit hard by these measures' high expenses. Not every facility can afford to have a spare set of tools on hand for every single process unit. Numerous innovations have been proposed, along with suggestions for new mechanisms to be put in place, to provide preventative technical maintenance for equipment [3–5].

DOI: 10.1201/9781003564904-6

An example of the strategy for planning pump maintenance for modern thermal power plants is described. Predicting future failures using the current operating parameters of the pumping equipment was done using a Weibull distribution model [6–10]. The study determined the optimal replacement interval for each component in the pumping system, taking into account system reliability in order to minimize the cost of redundant scheduled maintenance. The researchers addressed thermal power plant pump maintenance planning using data-driven reliability analysis.

This chapter presents a methodology for designing rotodynamic pump preventive maintenance systems with an emphasis on identifying anomalous occurrences associated with hydrodynamic operating circumstances. This technique is based on the features of the pump's experimental dynamic response to various loads and operational abnormalities. The method is used for a centrifugal pump of medium size. It has been shown that a diagnostic system may be built around basic decision criteria provided by spectrum evaluation of pressure signals recorded at the pump's intake or output [11].

Intelligent forecasting based on algorithms for neural networks and electronic centrifugal pump maintenance was introduced by the authors. It turns out that firms still have a hard time putting preventative maintenance approaches for pumps into reality, even though there have been a lot of studies on the topic. The majority of maintenance professionals at one hundred companies still just fix equipment when it breaks down, rather than focusing on preventative maintenance [12–15]. Moreover, many businesses that have developed programmes to execute preventative maintenance do not adhere to systematic procedures, as pointed out. So, it's clear that the research presents sophisticated answers to the problems that businesses experience when trying to execute preventative maintenance.

However, to evaluate the technical condition and service life of pumping equipment, the work associated with implementing the pump preventive maintenance system relies on the suggestions of collecting and processing big data, as well as implementing specific models and calculation complexes. Users or professionals operating this equipment collect all gathered data and transfer it for processing. One significant stumbling block to predictive analytics systems is the absence of a tool that can accurately identify the source of an issue or promptly identify a potentially hazardous scenario for the equipment. Consider the widespread belief that field maintenance data is not being used by technicians due to issues with data accessibility and dependability [16]. According to estimates, technicians devote over

13% of their overall maintenance time to researching and acquiring information for each piece of equipment. A programme that offers the correct information assistance for oil pump maintenance, together with enough computer support, may make these tasks easier. The authors of this article suggest employing an augmented reality system as such a tool.

The world is now experiencing the digitization era. Every industry and facet of human endeavour is being touched by the pervasive influence of digital technology. The researchers state that augmented reality is a high-quality digital tool for performing pump maintenance duties. Technicians may rely on the augmented reality system as their go-to decision-making tool by seamlessly integrating virtual and physical objects. Augmented reality systems have been used for equipment maintenance for some time. Systems like this are used, created, and demonstrated in a variety of research projects. An example of this would be the presentation of a literature review that summarizes the existing status of AR in service along with its most significant technical constraints [17–20]. The study's findings highlight the places that still need improvement. For instance, one of the primary obstacles to integrating AR technology into the business is the lack of standardized techniques for tracking and verifying their origin. It is challenging to draw comparisons between physical and digital items due to their inherent differences. The authors explored the possibility of using AR to build an oil industry–specific integrated object management system.

This research proposes a hybrid approach, integrating augmented reality with dynamic simulation. As a result, researchers can assess how well these technologies work together to maintain pumping equipment and come up with suggestions on how to improve, deploy, and work together with them. Dynamic modelling is based, to some extent, on the idea of digital twins.

The digital twin incorporates several functions, thus it is important to note that it's a complicated notion. To tackle local target objectives, for instance, one uses a numerical simulation system. This system employs a numerical simulation system that involves pumps and pump motors. The numerical simulation method is great for pinpointing certain problems, but it isn't enough when it comes to expanding functionality and tracking changes in technical parameters over time. A more appropriate technique here would be dynamic modelling.

To do this, the Methods and Materials section will outline how the dynamic model may be integrated with the virtual reality framework, and the procedures for carrying out experiments, testing, and assessing the system's efficacy will be provided. An application that combines augmented reality with dynamic simulation is described and built under the Experiments section. The Results and Discussion section presents an evaluation of the system's functionality, an analysis of the findings related to the development of the collaborative application, and the results of the experimental process. The recommendations for industrial companies on how to employ AR for oil pump servicing are laid out in Section 6.5.

6.2 METHODS AND MATERIALS

6.2.1 Main Augmented Reality System Functions

The primary goal of implementing an AR system into oil pump management is to provide a comprehensive platform for equipment functioning. When it comes to equipment maintenance, there are a lot of different methods to get the job done. These methods include contacting the dispatcher, looking for information on instruments, using paper or digital equipment manuals, and using third-party software. Logs of equipment maintenance are often maintained either manually or electronically, with little or no connection to the actual production site. To implement the aforementioned features, this study proposes an augmented reality system.

6.2.2 Improvements to the Dynamic Model's Framework and Its Interconnection with the AR Platform

This investigation made use of the separator model for oil flow separation. The model was created with the help of Aveva Dynamic Simulation. The authors stress that the model's creation and validation were not integral to this investigation but rather part of a different one. Several useful features were included in this model, which was connected with a server at the communication level. Consequently, the model might be integrated with an AR system and used together to enhance oil pump maintenance efficiency:

1. A process model, power system model, and automated system model were all part of the dynamic model, which served as an example;
2. Considering the facilities' inertia, the dynamic model predicted changes in technical parameters, energy supply system parameters, and automation system parameters;
3. The solver speed of the dynamic model was sufficient for real-time simulation. Use of this object in an AR system would allow for the delivery of object-related data in a reasonable amount of time;

4. The real-world object's sensors and actuators fed data into the dynamic device, which was then connected to the object's communication sheet;

5. The dynamic model's data changed at regular intervals, called "time steps." Data transmission techniques and the functioning of the network's communication layer dictated the size of the time step. The dynamic model continued to function normally regardless of the value of this time step. But at the level when the dynamic model was applied, it did impact the outcome.

A foundation for the development of a unique real-world virtual environment for the maintenance of pumping equipment has been established in this research. The features described in Section 6.2.1 are identical to those of the developed framework. Its adaptability and compatibility with various digital solutions and technologies, including analytical modules built on AI systems and digital twins, are key features. The protocols for data exchange between the system for augmented reality and the dynamic model were defined first. The OPC UA protocol is supported by Aveva Dynamic Simulation, which is the major integration protocol. The focus of this research was not the communication route that the designer of the interactive simulation software environment created between the dynamically generated model and the OPC server but instead discovering and validating a connection between the OPC server and the virtual reality system. It was difficult for the researchers to implement and configure the OPC UA in the environment for developing augmented reality applications. To get data from the OPC server, which the augmented-reality app uses in the same way as the web app, a dedicated polling block had to be built. This block would then pull the main code whenever it received data from the server. Due to the high probability of many mistakes caused by signal acquisition delays, the authors deemed this approach unsatisfactory. Figure 6.1 shows the suggested structure as a result.

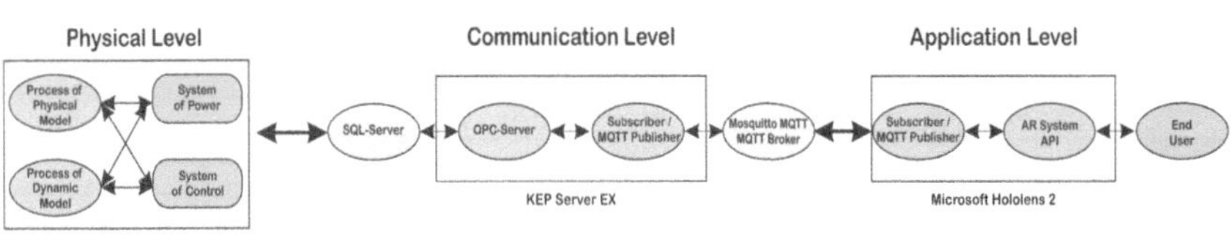

FIGURE 6.1 Results for suggested structure.

This framework relies on the use of the state-of-the-art MQTT protocol for data transmission. Incorporating the Mosquitto MQTT broker into the framework allowed for the coordination of transmitting messages between the AR system and the dynamic model. This protocol has been shown repeatedly to be a successful foundational protocol for IoT devices. The authors conclude that the following features and technical connections should be part of the ideal framework for creating a software application that combines dynamic simulation with an augmented reality system:

1. There are three tiers to the system: physical, application, and communication.
2. A fundamental structure of components, processes, and adaptable systems exists, with separate control and management systems. Systems are reclassified when maintenance increases. For production purposes, components may be relocated to real or online settings. If everything goes well, the systems work as intended. New algorithms are implemented using dynamic models in real or virtual control systems, decreasing commissioning and maintenance costs.
3. The messaging module mostly uses the MQTT and OPC protocols. With OPC, the power supply system, automation system, and dynamic model may all talk to one another. After that, the OPC server posts its data to the MQTT agent, which in turn communicates with the HoloLens 2 AR software. The SQL server acts as a tool to record any changes made at any level in this structure. There are timestamps associated with each value. All parts must be in sync with one another in terms of time if the system is to function properly.
4. The system's physical and communication layers are structured in a manner that allows it to be linked to any system that uses digital technologies. Just being able to communicate data using both the MQTT/OPC protocols is enough.
5. The architecture emphasizes the HoloLens 2 augmented reality software at the application level. It should be mentioned that a user-interface device might be a smartphone or tablet. There will be no disruption to the solution's core operation, but the advanced features of the HoloLens 2 application, particularly those about the 3D visualization method and others, need to be highlighted.

6.2.3 The Experimental Procedures, Validation, and Assessment of the System's Performance

The process of testing and assessing the system's efficacy is fraught with complexity and uncertainty. There needs to be much more research on this procedure and problem. The authors stress that this is a pioneering study on the topic of complicated augmented reality methods for oil pump maintenance, which means that testing will be much easier. Testing should become increasingly involved as development progresses towards completion, with the creation of a dedicated testing application and the execution of algorithms at various levels of the system's architecture.

6.3 EXPERIMENTAL SETUP

Figure 6.2 shows the apparatus in the lab, which included a Grundfos electric motor-powered vertical centrifugal pump. This pump was used as a service item.

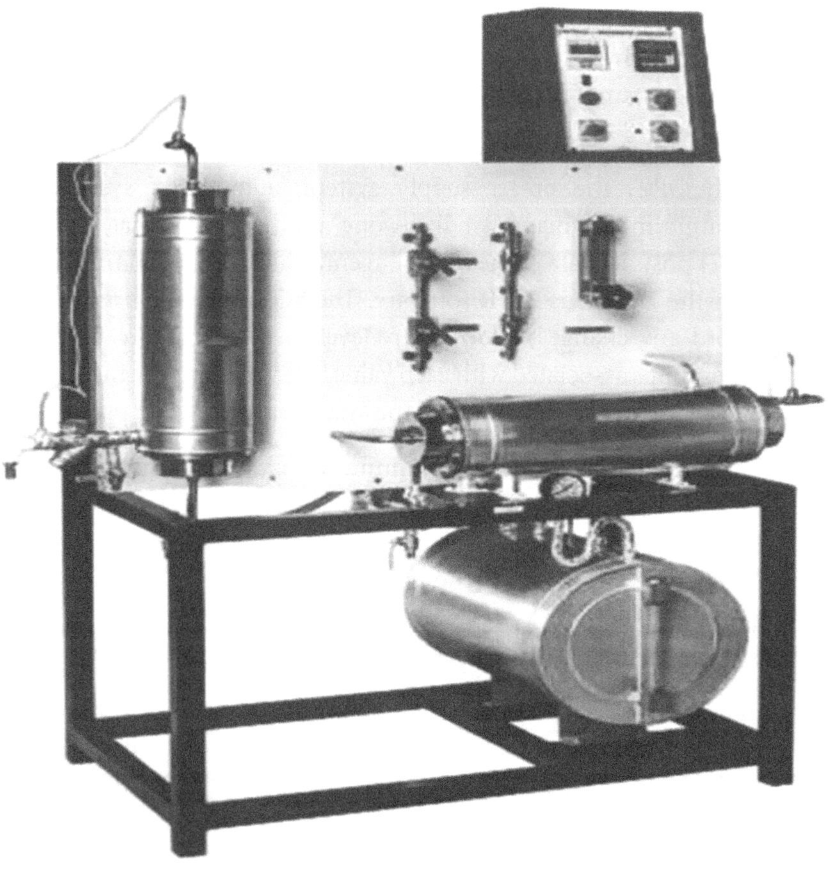

FIGURE 6.2 Laboratory setup.

The installation's equipment featured two Grundfos pumps, a heat exchanger, a pipeline portion, controls, sensors, and electric actuators, as well as two tanks. Various indications, including supply, pressure, temperature, and pressure decrease, were shown by the sensors. The power supply system's physical simulation hub is shown in Figure 6.3, and the power system's control system's physical simulation hub is shown in Figure 6.4.

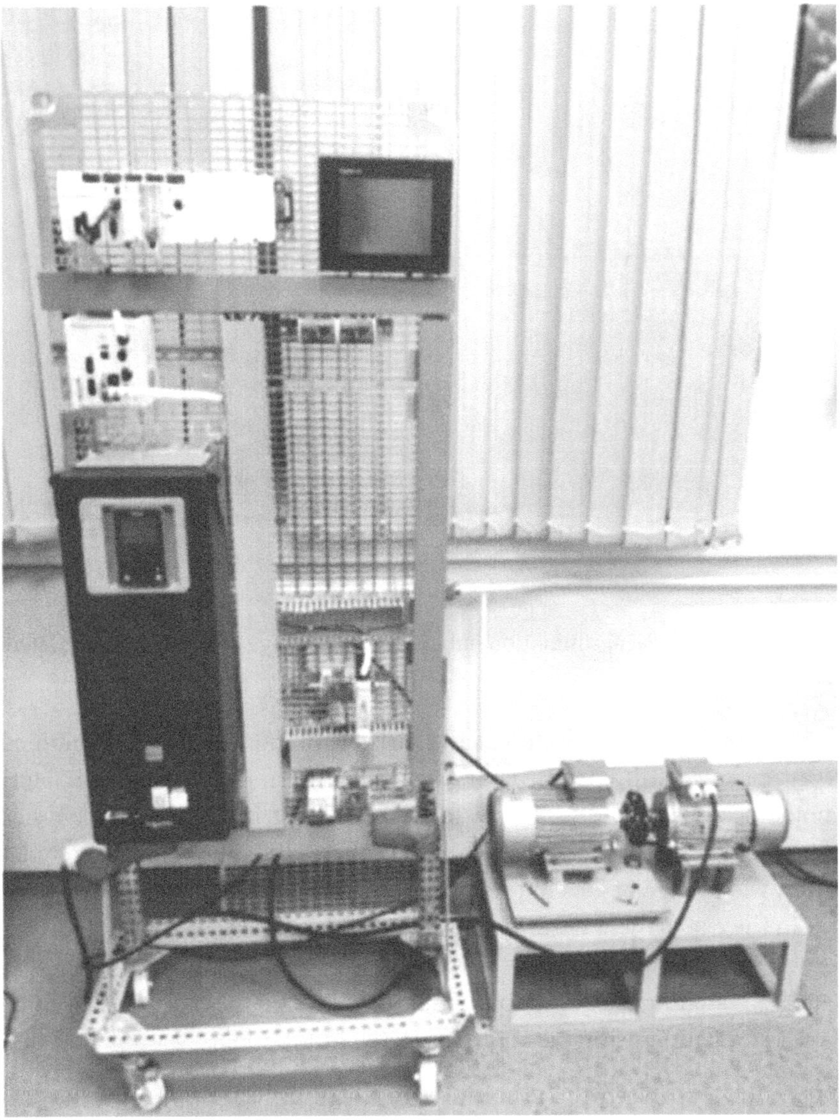

FIGURE 6.3 Physical simulation hub for the power supply system.

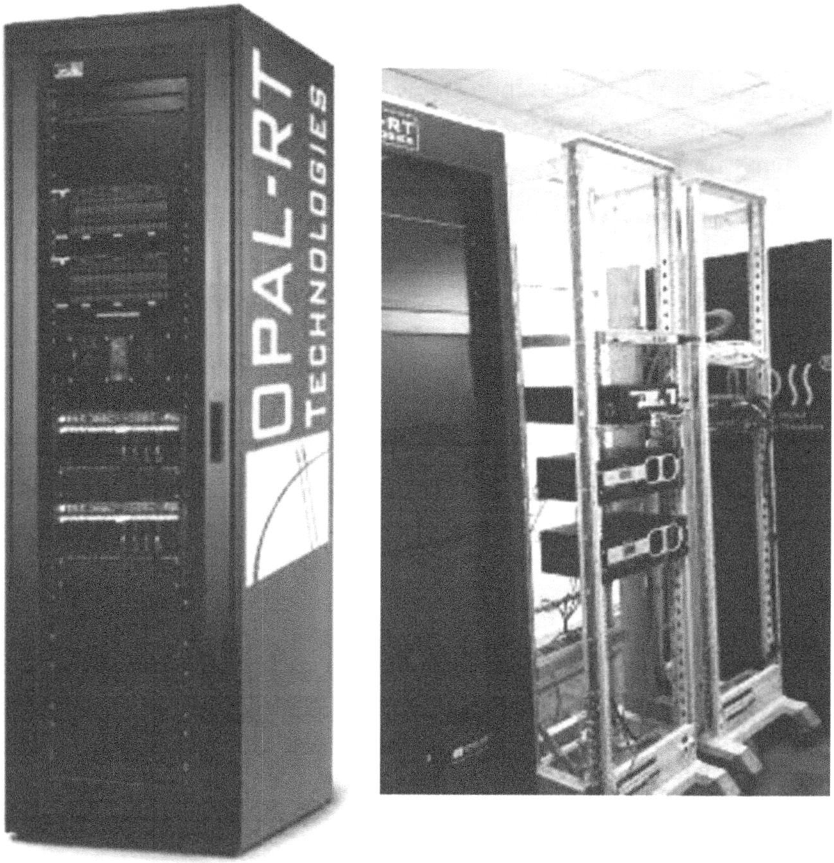

FIGURE 6.4 Physical simulation hub for the control system of the power system.

The joint usage of the actual and virtual components of the equipment was the key distinguishing characteristic of the applied equipment. Here, both the control and power systems could exist in a virtual or physical form. Users might move freely between these different systems, completing a wide range of jobs in the process.

In the experiment described in this chapter,

1. An augmented reality pump maintenance application with dynamic simulation using the approach stated in Section 6.2.2 was developed.
2. The team used the procedures outlined in Section 6.2.3 to test the software.

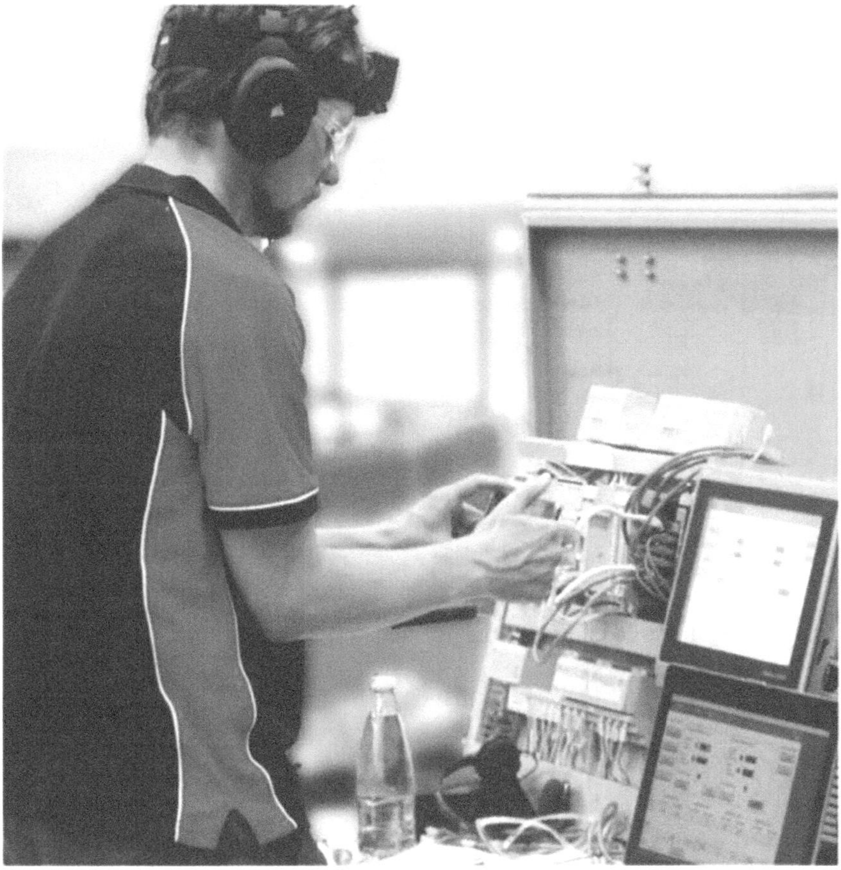

FIGURE 6.5 Generated software's testing procedure.

Microsoft HoloLens 2 glasses were used for interaction by users with the AR technology. The generated software's testing procedure is shown in Figure 6.5.

6.4 RESULTS AND DISCUSSION

This application was developed in Unity software to evaluate the efficacy of the methods presented in the chapter. An enlarged image of the finished app can be seen in Figure 6.6. There was no difference between the dynamic model and the 3D installation model. From the dynamic model to the data channels to the communication server and beyond, the variable names remained consistent. Consistently naming tags was crucial since it cut down on development time and mistakes. The OPC Quick

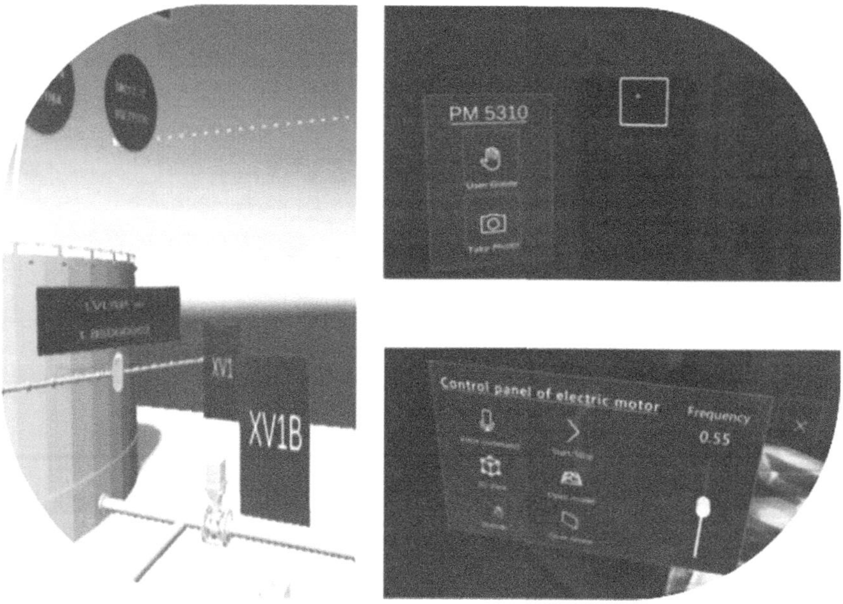

FIGURE 6.6 Enlarged image of the finished app.

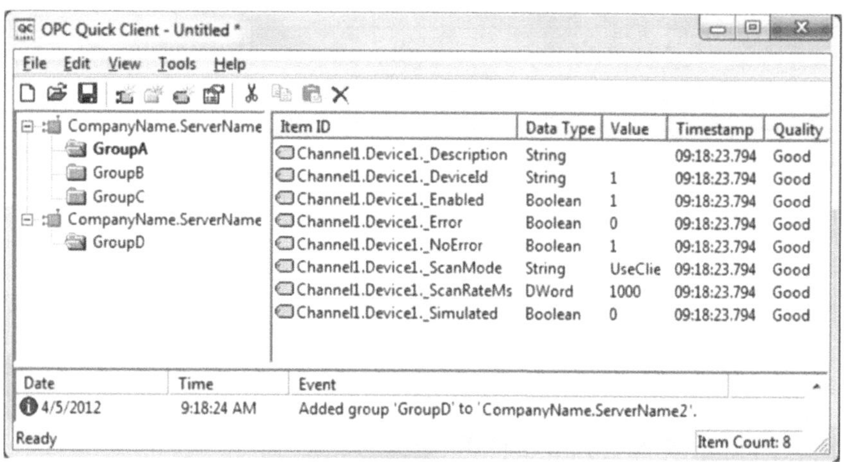

FIGURE 6.7 OPC Quick Client's dynamic model variables.

Client's dynamic model variables used to build Application 1 are shown in Figure 6.7.

The MQTT broker is shown in Figure 6.8. The KEPServer agent received data via the Aveva OPC servers and sent it to the Mosquito brokerage. The subject IoT Aveva was subscribed to by the agent. By subscribing to the IoT

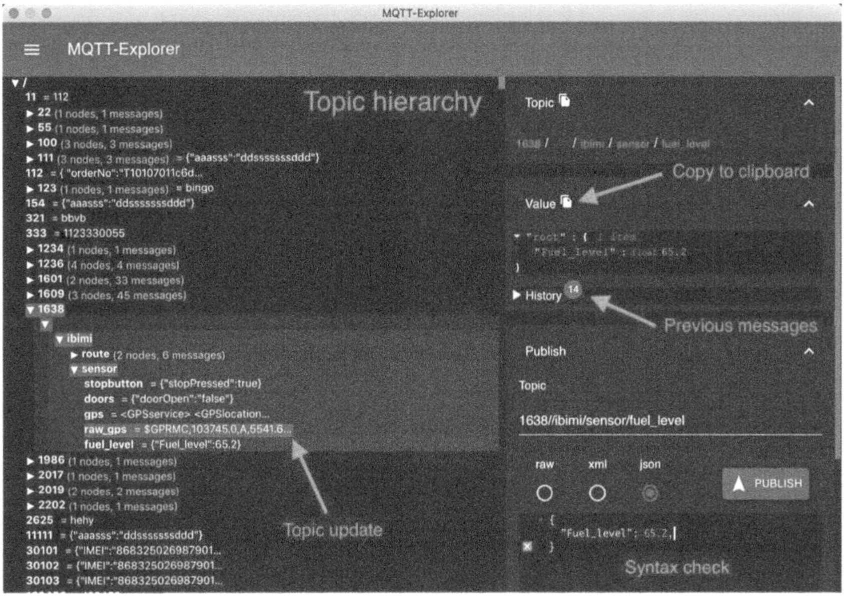

FIGURE 6.8 MQTT broker.

gateway topic, the MQTT agent sent user messages to the broker over the MQTT AR system. Furthermore, the OPC server received data from the MQTT broker using the MQTT client KEP server, which was subscribed to this subject.

To test how well the dynamic model and augmented reality system worked together, three apps were created. The 3D model represents one installation with fifteen parameters, two of which are adjustable. These parameters could be modified in several ways: (1) at any level of the system; (2) with an augmented reality app; (3) with three units identical to the installation in point (1); and (4) with five units identical to the installation in point (1). The appearance of tested system is shown in Figure 6.9, with the image acquired through the live broadcast of the Microsoft HoloLens application.

Consequently, there were three sections of the laboratory. Researchers were able to link the first to the power supply system via a technical procedure involving pumps, and the second to it through a power system simulation unit that housed some of the energy-mechanical equipment, such as pump motors with control systems and smart shields. The primary technical variables, including stress, flow rate, and temperature, were measured at various locations on the laboratory apparatus. Power supply systems

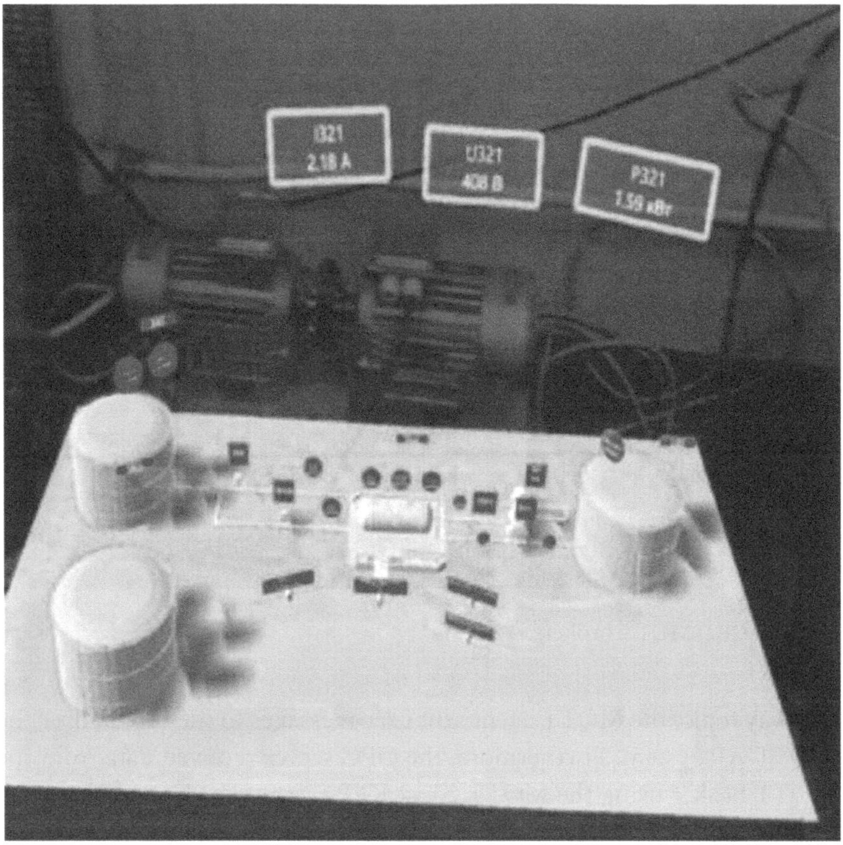

FIGURE 6.9 Tested system's appearance.

and technological process co-modelling are shown in the dynamic model. In the laboratory unit, they could see some of the actual equipment. An example of this would be a pump motor equipped with smart shield switches and sensors for power, voltage, and current. Researchers made it possible to regulate the power supply.

This apparatus stood in for actual objects. Their three-dimensional representations showed not just the same objects but also other objects in a dynamic model. Figure 6.9 displays the comprehensive 3D representation of the installation. In addition to providing a three-dimensional image of the installation, the app illustrated the real-time adjustment of the dynamic model's parameters. Figure 6.1 shows that this allowed for creation of both a dynamic process model and physical representations of its components. A more in-depth industrial 3D model of the installation shows how the user interacts with the equipment through the augmented reality system.

The equipment is represented by a dynamic model and its 3D image, and the user can use the control buttons and laboratory stands to read control signals and change the machinery's actual condition. The reason for this is because Figure 6.8 displays a list of potential variables for the dynamic model. Its tag names were set by the makers of the Aveva Dynamic Simulations programme and generated automatically. The unit's collected variables are labelled in Figure 6.9, which matches the industrial object's labelling. The parameters of automation systems, energy systems, augmented reality applications, dynamic models, and parameters often found in industrial organizations were incompatible. The variable name must adhere to a certain standard. The variables are linked together using specific linking tables, although, at the moment, no such standards are in use.

The dynamic model was refined by removing the following variables: those related to the specialized automation system's operation; the predetermined point feed for temperature variations; the flow in streams as well as equipment; the pressure, temperature, and flow rate in the raw streams, the source, the drum, and the final reservoirs. Additional power system characteristics were recorded, including the positions of valves XV1 XV2, XV3, and XV4 as well as the statuses of motors M1, M3, and M4. An example list of these variables is shown in Figure 6.8. It is possible to show any system parameter if needed. The production name is shown with the engine variables in Figure 6.9. To ensure ease of recognition for users, standard naming conventions were used: I321 for current, U321 for voltage, and P321 for power.

Figure 6.10 displays the results of the NASA-TLX exam, which evaluates the application's cognitive and psychological aspects.

This figure displays the mean NASA-TLX test scores of all individuals who took part in the study. The study had 93 participants in total. There were 81 men and 17 women who took part, with ages ranging from 21 to 28. Five distinct scenarios of "pump failure detected by vibration sensors" were modelled to implement the test. The mission was to turn off the pump. The participants were divided into groups, following these steps:

1. The only tools available to the testers were smart shielding and the ability to contact someone who had access to the equipment;
2. All system promoter values may be examined by the testers using a smart shield as well as a SCADA system;
3. The testers were provided with a smart shield as well as paperwork that detailed the system's connection process;

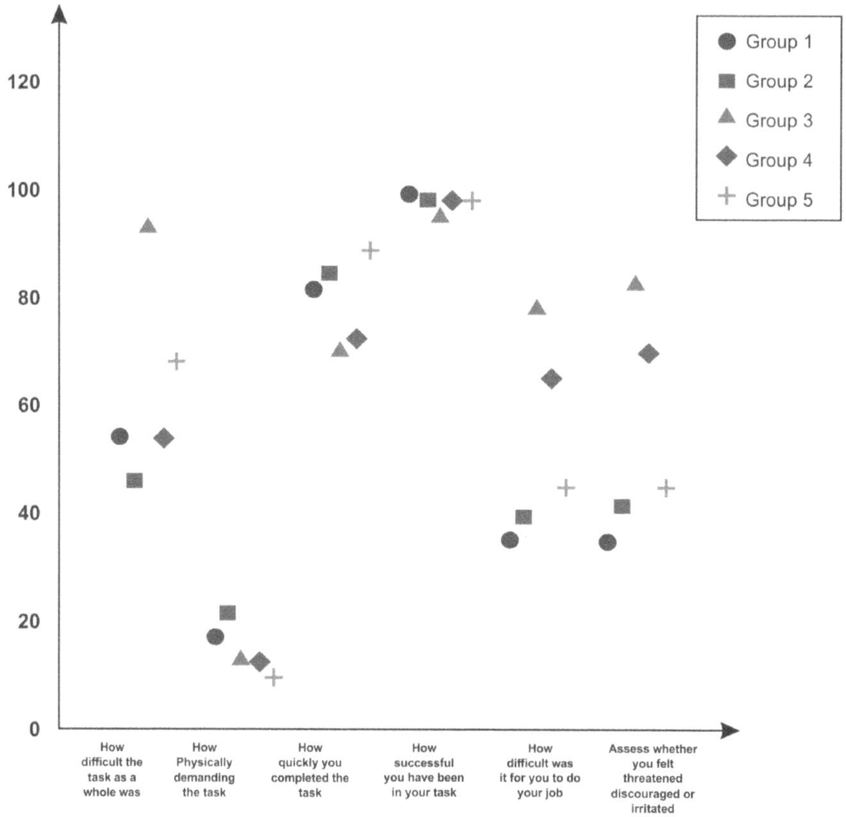

FIGURE 6.10 Results of the NASA-TLX exam.

4. The only way to interact was via augmented reality technology, and orders had to be input by hand;
5. Voice or physical input was the sole means of command, and the only means of interaction was the augmented reality system.

According to the findings, the test subjects reported feeling less endangered when using the AR system but felt burdened by the task's complexity and its perceived importance. They did, however, make notice of the task's physical difficulty. This was likely caused by the need to engage with the AR goggles to a great extent. The trials were conducted in student groups; thus, it is important to note that the participants' ages were all under 27. In a professional or corporate setting, this average age would likely be higher. Consequently, it would be beneficial to include a new metric for the degree of skill in using AR goggles as part of the system's performance evaluation. Most of the people who tested the glasses in this article had never used them before, therefore their expertise was severely lacking.

6.5 CONCLUSION

In this study, researchers show that it is possible and beneficial to use AR and dynamic modelling together to perform oil pump maintenance. Here are the main points: (1) A centralized communication layer that transports data via protocols such as OPC UA and MQTT should be a part of the system, and it should be portable and scalable. (2) Using precise 3D and dynamic models, the modular architecture should allow for the replacement of physical pieces with virtual ones to enhance functionality. (3) It is important to examine the application's performance as well as its cognitive and psychological implications. (4) The system demonstrated no noticeable deterioration in performance when tested with up to five interactive models. (5) Cognitive testing showed that when performing emergency shutdown activities, there were improvements in physical and mental demands, time pressure, performance, and frustration. The research also lays out plans for the future, including investigating the potential industrial uses of virtual twins along with additional digital technologies, expanding dynamic models, and incorporating diagnostic equipment for oil pumps' life-cycle assessment.

REFERENCES

1. Rathore, P. S., S. Ahuja, S. R. Burri, A. Khunteta, A. Baliyan, & A. Kumar, (2024). *Deep learning techniques for automation and industrial applications.* John Wiley & Sons, Inc.; Scrivener Publishing LLC.
2. Hampiholi, Narayan. "Elevating emergency healthcare-technological advancements and challenges in smart ambulance systems and advanced monitoring and diagnostic tools." *International Journal of Computer Trends and Technology* 72.1 (2024): 1–7.
3. Cheng, Ruijie, Lei Hou, and Sheng Xu. "A review of digital twin applications in civil and infrastructure emergency management." *Buildings* 13.5 (2023): 1143.
4. Preethi, D., and R. S. Valarmathi. "AR/VR and robotics and their role in leadership." In R. Geetha, Nhu-Ngoc Dao, Saeed Khalid (eds) *Impact of New Technology on Next-Generation Leadership.* IGI Global, 2024. 162–178.
5. Wagner, Paul, and Dalal Alharthi. "Leveraging VR/AR/MR/XR technologies to improve cybersecurity education, training, and operations." *Journal of Cybersecurity Education, Research and Practice* 2024.1 (2023): 7.
6. Rane, Nitin. "Role of ChatGPT and similar generative artificial intelligence (AI) in the construction industry." Available at SSRN 4598258 (2023). https://papers.ssrn.com/sol3/papers.cfm?abstract_id=4598258

7. Kumar, T. R., G. Laxmaiah, and S. S. Raj. "A framework of intelligent manufacturing process by integrating various functions." In Deepa Jose, Preethi Nanjundan, Sanchita Paul, Sachi Nandan Mohanty (eds) *AI-Driven IoT Systems for Industry 4.0*. CRC Press. 241–254, 2024.
8. Birtill, Michael, et al. "The use of immersive simulation in paramedicine education: a scoping review." *Interactive Learning Environments* 31.4 (2023): 2428–2443.
9. Mewada, Shivlal, et al. "Smart diagnostic expert system for a defect in forging process by using machine learning process." *Journal of Nanomaterials* 2022.1 (2022): 2567194.
10. Almessabi, Hanan, and Mousa Al-Fairy. "Unlocking the future of farming: a review of metaverse integration in agriculture." *IEEE Engineering Management Review* 53.3, (2024): 128–143.
11. Tsaknaki, Electra, et al. *XR-state of play, market needs, training trends*. Dissertation. ERASMUS-EDU-2023-PI-ALL-INNO., 2024.
12. Kumar, T. Rajasanthosh, Kesaraju Venkata Sai Pavan, Rajesh Kukati, and Mandala Srinivasa Reddy. "Quantitatively examines the feasibility of different configurations of the aftermarket supply chain enabling additive manufacturing." *Solid State Technology* 63.5 (2020): 492–507.
13. Agrawal, Rashmi, Pramod Singh Rathore, Ganesh Gopal Deverajan, and Rajiva Ranjan Divivedi, eds. *Artificial Intelligence and Cybersecurity in Healthcare*. John Wiley & Sons, 2025. https://www.scrivenerpublishing.com/cart/title.php?id=1101
14. Zafar, Muhammad Hamza, Even Falkenberg Langås, and Filippo Sanfilippo. "Exploring the synergies between collaborative robotics, digital twins, augmentation, and industry 5.0 for smart manufacturing: a state-of-the-art review." *Robotics and Computer-Integrated Manufacturing* 89 (2024): 102769.
15. Cabanes, Ria Valerie D., et al. "Issues, innovations, and challenges: simulation technologies in related learning experiences." *SN Computer Science* 5.5 (2024): 613.
16. Trivedi, Shantanu, and Saurabh Tiwari. "The resurgence of augmented reality and virtual reality in construction: past, present, and future directions." *Augmented and Virtual Reality in Industry* 5.2 (2023): 275.
17. Chen, Zhengyi, Keyu Chen, and Jack C. P. Cheng. "ISM-based analysis of VR-AEC adoption barriers and their inner mechanisms." *Engineering Construction and Architectural Management* 30.9 (2023): 4271–4293.
18. Wilkins, Holly Vanessa, et al. "Application of augmented reality for crime scene investigation training and education." *Science & Justice* 64.3 (2024): 289–296.
19. de Lurdes Calisto, Maria, and Soumodip Sarkar. "A systematic review of virtual reality in tourism and hospitality: the known and the paths to follow." *International Journal of Hospitality Management* 116 (2024): 103623.
20. Pedram, Shiva, Grace Kennedy, and Sal Sanzone. "Toward the validation of VR-HMDs for medical education: a systematic literature review." *Virtual Reality* 27.3 (2023): 2255–2280.

CHAPTER 7

Integrating Virtual Reality into Disaster Response Training

V.S.N. Murthy, K. Suresh Kumar, Harinadh Karimikonda, and Kiran Sree Pokkuluri

7.1 INTRODUCTION

The risks of disasters are on the rise in many regions of our more interconnected globe due to factors including irresponsible urban planning, environmental degradation, and ineffective leadership. The current tendency of corporate and public investments to disregard catastrophe risks greatly increases the likelihood of future losses. Investments in disaster education and micro-level mitigation methods are part of this category. Making people more self-sufficient and disaster-ready is the key to preventing this major threat to social welfare and economic progress. It is the duty of educational institutions to effectively communicate the procedures that should be followed in the event of an emergency.

In earlier times, trainees learned about safety using more traditional means, such as in-person sessions, written materials (such as procedure safety manuals and brochures), or online modules with easy-to-understand questions. Most of these ways of presenting information are fine in theory, but how successful they really are is debatable. There are many degrees and types of learning, according to Dale's study on the use of audio-visual technologies in the classroom. This is an example of how Dale demonstrated that learning is mostly dependent on practical application and experience,

DOI: 10.1201/9781003564904-7

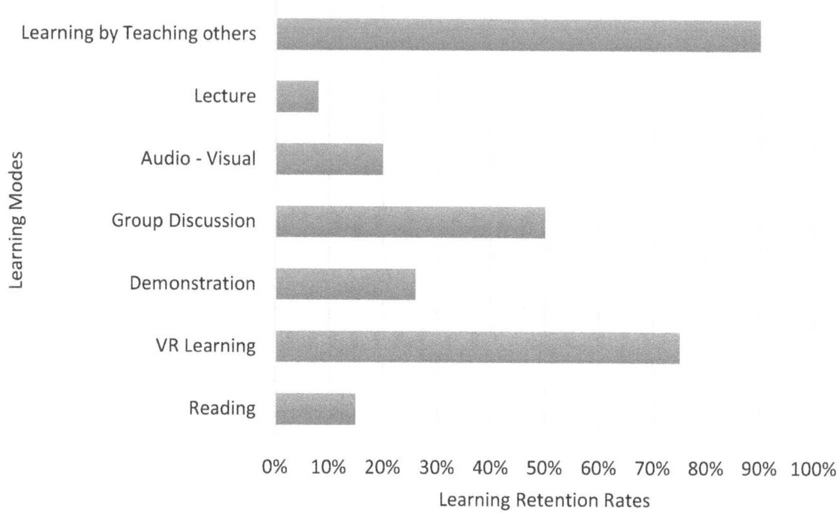

FIGURE 7.1 Comparing learning retention rates across modes.

rather than relying just on theoretical explanations conveyed in books, videos, or audio recordings. Figure 7.1 indicates that direct experience and applied learning provide the strongest support.

Several new avenues for cutting-edge educational and training possibilities have opened up thanks to virtual reality technology. Among the many potential technological advancements are the following: the ability to immerse oneself in a virtual environment in real time, allowing learners to virtually interact with and imagine a three-dimensional representation; the ability to enhance one's conceptual understanding through the creation or modification of digital simulations; the visualization of random ideas; the dynamic visualization of correlations among numerous factors in a virtual system; the freedom to experience three-dimensional space from any angle; and the ability to access and participate in events and locations that would otherwise be impractical or prohibitively expensive, dangerous, or otherwise impractical to visit in person. Virtual reality has various uses in education and, when used properly, may have a favourable effect on learning because of its possibilities, some of which are exclusive to this technology [1–3].

7.2 RELATED WORKS

Industrial professionals, delegates from multinational corporations, and various NGOs, along with instructors, attended the conference held in Indian university of management. The main objective of this conference was to compile and review the issues in demand forecasting and logistics operations happening in humanitarian programmes. Providing training on operational procedures procedures to these humanitarian organisations is essential. As a result, the instructors are in constant research seeking an efficient way for training and implementing it in the field. Likewise, recognizing the importance of training to this generation of disaster response teams, both the team members and the team as a whole are subsequently evaluated on how they could improve performance and outcomes.

With the help of this conference, participants are able to analyse the main issue being held in humanitarian organisations and disaster management organisations. The problems are classified from lacking skills to deformity of funds. The lack of skill and training appears to be a bigger issue because of language barriers, poor staff management, and personnel moving on to more productive jobs. These challenges became more critical because of limited resources and inconsistent funding. Convincing institutional investors to support skill development and training programs for disaster response teams is difficult due to their lack of trust in the effectiveness of such initiatives. However, there is a shortage of qualified trainers who have enough knowledge or practical experience, as well as a lack of theoretical materials related to this field [4].

At the same university, a study was conducted among 30 students whowere equally divided into two groups to explore the effectiveness of experiential and applied learning through virtual reality simulators. The students were assigned to Group A or Group B. Group A students wore virtual reality headsets that fully immersed them in the simulation environment, while Group B experienced the same simulation on a standard computer monitor.

Both groups interacted with the simulation using controllers and gaming pads. The results showed improved knowledge and skills regarding the simulation they played; however, Group A showed significantly greater improvement than Group B because of the immersive nature of the VR headsets. Hence, this study shows how learning through virtual reality simulation enhances skills of the team and especially when it is used through VR headsets [5, 6].

7.3 SUGGESTED DESIGN

Several factors necessitated the use of gamification into this project (Figure 7.2). Research shows that students are more engaged and enthusiastic when presented with game-like scenarios rather than dry text or

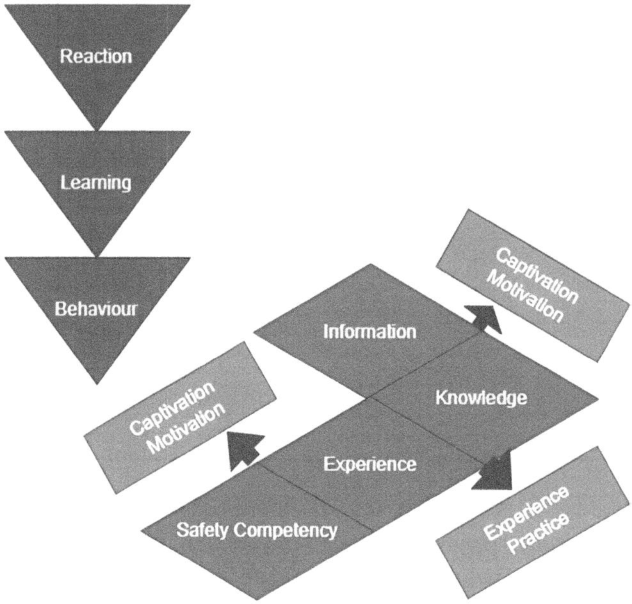

FIGURE 7.2 Suggested design framework.

one-on-one instruction. Training that is as realistic as may help the student better cope with the emotional shock of an emergency by strengthening their memoryretention and incorporating intuitive learning.

The initiative takes the shape of a video game where the participant (henceforth called trainee) dons a virtual reality headset and pretends to be a character dealing with a particular catastrophe. The player character starts off in a basic setting, such an office building, that has just been or is about to be affected by an emergency, like a fire. The trainee is allowed some flexibility to handle things their own way; if they succeed, the simulation would tell us whether they survived the emergency and if they helped any of their virtual fellow victims. For example, a disaster may ensue if the trainee uses the elevator during a fire [7].

In addition to informing the trainee of typical dangers caused by disinformation, the scenario includes realistically placed interactive items that the character may employ to boost their odds of survival. A variety of fire extinguishers are provided in the fire scenario, along with operating instructions. A danger notice is included to advise against using water-based extinguishers on flames that have been ignited electrically [8].

The majority of the items in the simulation player's field of view are non-interactive and only serve to heighten the player's immersion in the catastrophe, but a small number of them are interactive and controllable by the player. Although the inclusion of additional interactive items enhances the realism of the catastrophe by providing more variables, it also expands the simulation's breadth, making control more difficult and diminishing the intended instruction.

The game is designed to raise awareness of safety measures in an interactive fashion by drawing from real-life conventions and regulations. At each stage of the scenario, the player will be presented with numerous choices. Some of these choices will be based on safety rules, while others will reflect frequent errors that someone could make due to trauma or ignorance of the protocols [9, 10]. This is all part of the current execution plan. Following this, the trainee virtual character's actions will have either positive or negative outcomes. As a result, the trainees internalize knowledge on both what to do and what not to do in the event of an emergency.

7.4 METHODS AND PROCEDURES

This simulation was built using Unreal Engine 4, an open-source gaming engine that allows for integrated modelling, texturing, scripting, and gameplay design. The engine's support for C++ programming makes it easy to create in-game objects with a variety of features that may inherit from one another and create unique environments. For example, the scenario depicts a world where many items, such as fabric and tables, may transform into fire when near a flame (Figure 7.3a–c).

7.4.1 Designing the Layout

A standard office building is shown in the first scenario. A number of office buildings' architectural plans were examined in order to extract commonalities; they included elevators, furnished conference rooms, lobby areas, fire escapes, and so on. Use of universal signs and symbols, such as those seen on fire extinguishers and fire exits, serves as a guiding reference in the simulation. As a result, it is easier to overcome the language barrier and become familiar with symbols.

The office floor was created using the unreal editor, which is capable of turning static polygons into materials for desired constructions. Rooms are furnished with things like lights, furniture, and more to help distinguish the layout from its fundamental structure.

There is more than one method to engage with some of these objects. This encompasses anything from furniture that may catch fire to the canisters of fire extinguishers that are used to put out particular areas of fire so that people can escape.

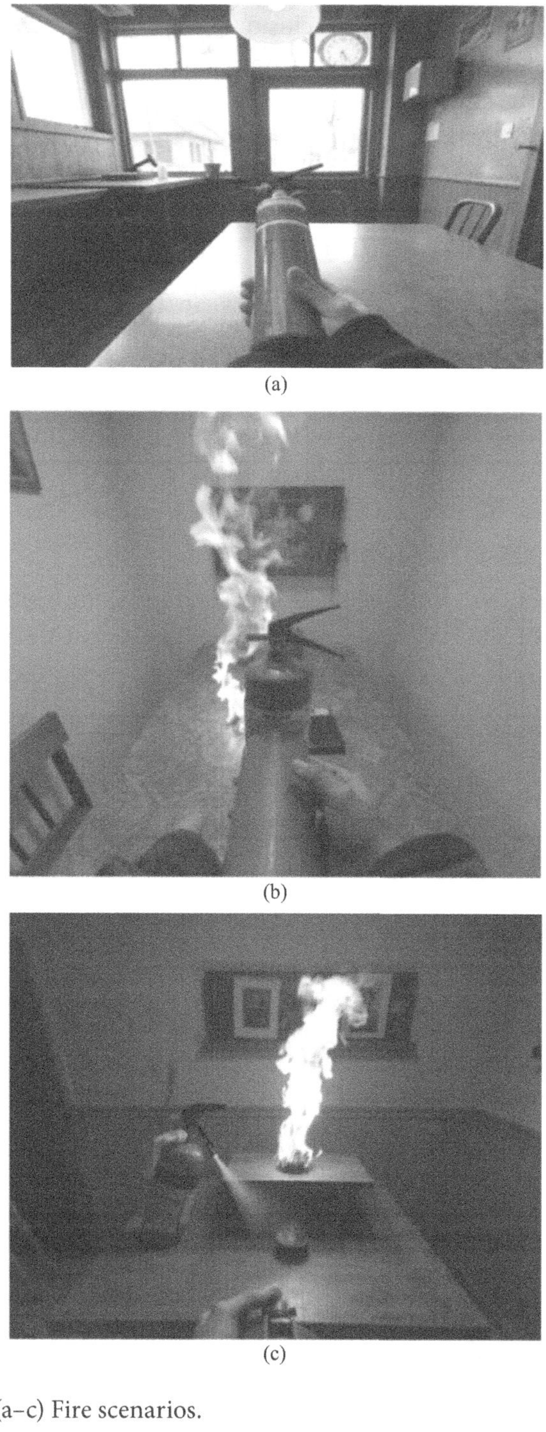

FIGURE 7.3 (a–c) Fire scenarios.

7.4.2 The Character Controller

The learner has the option to put themselves in the shoes of the character and see the world through their eyes in the simulation. A gamepad linked to the Android handset using Bluetooth controls the character's movement. One button lets the user crouch, another allows interaction with nearby objects like a fire extinguisher, and the movement options include forward, backward, left, and right (Figure 7.4). The simulation also makes use of head tracking, which means that the trainee's field of vision will shift in response to head movements, using the gyro sensor integrated into the android smartphone [11–13].

7.4.3 Interactive Elements

The interactive elements consist of objects that can catch on fire, fire extinguishers, and elevators. It is diagrammatically displayed in Figure 7.5.

7.4.3.1 Objects with Potential to Catch Fire

The learner must adapt to or avoid the shifting environment to make the simulation more realistic. Assuming the first scenario, the ecosystem burns down gradually. There is a common class for all things that may catch fire and have comparable characteristics. The visual asset, flammability, and distance at which an object may catch fire are all attributes of that item [14, 15]. The visual asset is in charge of how the item looks; it might be anything from a

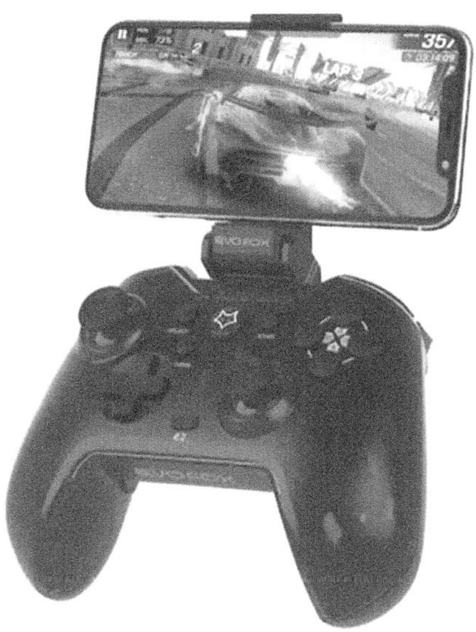

FIGURE 7.4 Character controller.

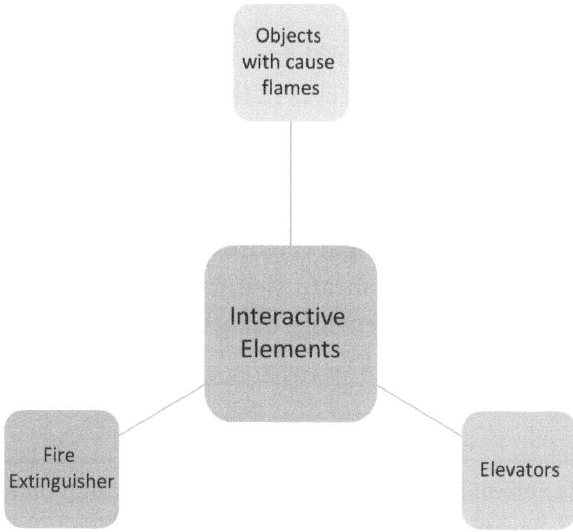

FIGURE 7.5 Interactive elements.

chair to some drapes. A material's flammability dictates how quickly it burns when it comes into contact with another material's flames, while its range specifies the furthest distance another item may be from it before it can catch fire. Algorithm 7.1 controls the spread of fire.

ALGORITHM 7.1 CONTROLS THE SPREAD OF FIRE

```
#include <iostream>
using namespace std;
 structFire()
 {
  for.on class = Bool;
  class in range = true;
  Object _ array[]return in object range (for);
  else each (object obj in _ array)
 }
  obj.Fire();
 {
  if else
 }
 {
  class in range<0>1+1;
  Intensity--0;
  }while (return.for)
```

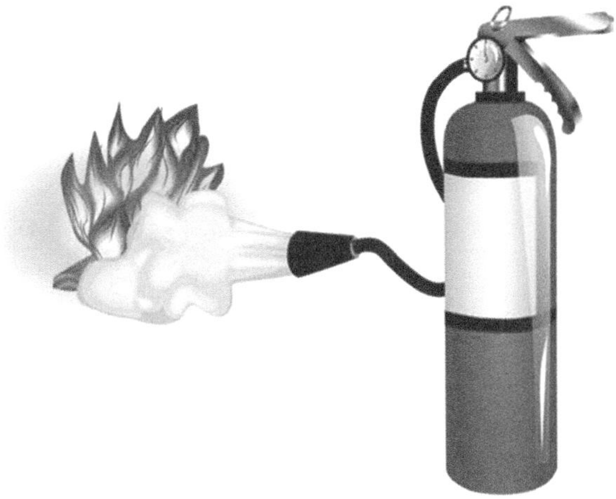

FIGURE 7.6 Fire extinguisher.

7.4.3.2 Fire Extinguisher

As a matter of safety practice, the majority of buildings contain a variety of fire extinguishers (Figure 7.6): Types A, B, C, D, and E. The simulation makes an effort to include most of them while demonstrating how each one may be put to use. All the different kinds of extinguishers belong to the same class. To physically differentiate them, they share attributes like type-tag and visual asset. To account for the fact that various extinguishers provide different outcomes when used in the same situation, the remaining functions are type based.

7.4.3.3 Elevators

The simulation uses elevators to emphasize the message, even though everyone knows they shouldn't be utilized in a fire. An integral aspect of the simulation's dynamic setting is the elevator [16, 17]. The elevator may be summoned from any level and ridden, but the visual clues of smoke in the shaft indicate the risk of asphyxia. Once the trainee boards the lift, the process stops and the smoke in the shaft increases [18–25]. Then, the student must restart the simulation from an earlier point (Figure 7.7).

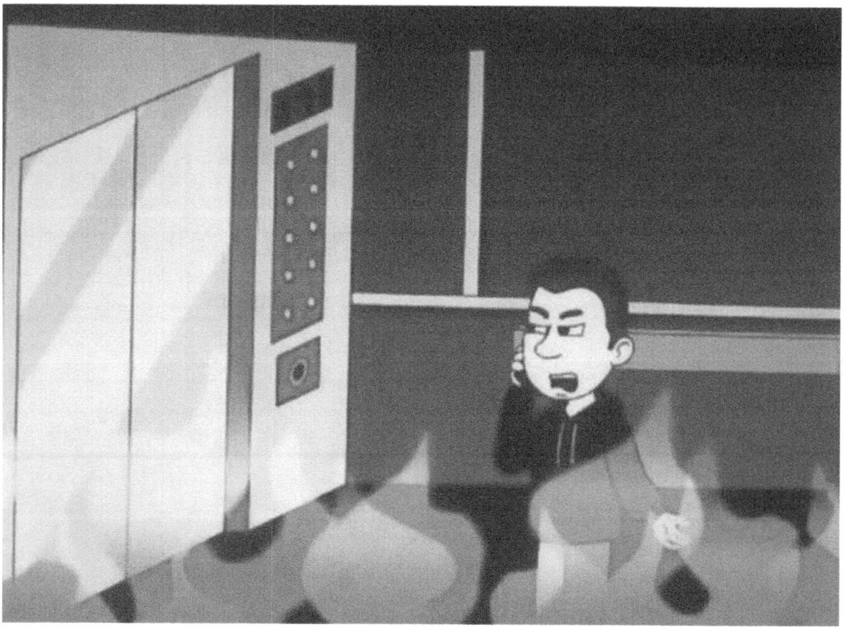

FIGURE 7.7 Elevator.

7.5 CONCLUSION

In conclusion, virtual reality is a state-of-the-art area with promising applications in many other sectors, and researchers are actively investigating these possibilities. Virtual reality is quickly becoming a popular and potentially game-changing tool in the field of safety training, among its many other potential uses. The need for creative, scalable, and efficient training solutions is growing in importance as the way humans engage with technologies and the environment changes. Virtual reality is showing to be more than a fad; it's a potent tool that will remain and influence training in the years to come. Construction, manufacturing, healthcare, and aviation are just a few of the many sectors that have shown interest in virtual reality safety training. Thanks to virtual reality's engrossing nature, users may safely experience realistic, high-risk events. Not only does this kind of training assist employees to gain practical skills, but it also improves their confidence and efficiency when responding to real-life situations. Virtual reality's capacity to provide engaging, repeatable, and cost-effective learning experiences is what distinguishes it from more conventional safety training techniques. Using these simulations, trainees may experience things that would be very difficult, if not impossible, or extremely expensive to do in real life. Virtual reality training also has the added benefit of being adaptable to the demands of each learner, allowing for a more customized learning experience. Virtual reality's potential applications in safety training are almost endless. There are a vast variety of potential uses for virtual reality technology, from studying first aid and operating heavy equipment to conducting emergency response exercises and identifying hazards. Virtual reality's growing use in safety training bodes well for the future, opening up novel avenues for educating employees to meet the unique hazards of their jobs. Virtual reality is crucial to safety instruction, not simply entertainment. It can transform safety procedure instruction into something more entertaining, effective, and accessible. As the technology grows more accessible and pervasive, VR will become a staple of security training programs worldwide, creating more secure work environments and more competent, confident workers. Safety training using virtual reality is not only an invention; it's a vital step towards preparing people for a complicated and high-risk future.

REFERENCES

1. Ahmadi, Maryam, Saied Yousefi, and Atie Ahmadi. "Exploring the most effective feedback system for training people in earthquake emergency preparedness using immersive virtual reality serious games." *International Journal of Disaster Risk Reduction* 110 (2024): 104630.
2. Yu, Xinhua, et al. "Integrating virtual reality and building information modeling for improving highway tunnel emergency response training." *Buildings* 12.10 (2022): 1523.
3. Khanal, Shishir, et al. "Virtual and augmented reality in the disaster management technology: a literature review of the past 11 years." *Frontiers in Virtual Reality* 3 (2022): 843195.
4. Alshowair, Abdulmajeed, et al. "Use of virtual reality exercises in disaster preparedness training: a scoping review." *SAGE Open Medicine* 12 (2024): 20503121241241936.
5. Keya, Rashika Tasnim, Ilona Helda, Tord Hettervik Frgland, Orsolya Székely-Keresztesi, Zoltán Székely, and Espen Kon. "Emergency Preparedness Training Using Virtual Reality Games: Allowing Knowledge Transfer in the Digital Age." In *European Conference on Knowledge Management*, pp. 369–378. Academic Conferences International Limited, 2024.
6. Shujuan, Liao, et al. "The use of virtual reality to improve disaster preparedness among nursing students: a randomized study." *Journal of Nursing Education* 61.2 (2022): 93–96.
7. Kumar, T. Rajasanthosh, et al. "Implementation of intelligent CPS for integrating the industry and manufacturing process." In Deepa Jose, Preethi Nanjundan, Sanchita Paul, Sachi Nandan Mohanty (eds) *AI-Driven IoT Systems for Industry 4.0*. CRC Press, 2024. 273–288.

8. Kimura, Ryohei, et al. "Scoping review of virtual reality (VR)-based disaster mitigation education." *Cureus* 16.11 (2024): e74062.
9. Sivakumar, S., R. Raffik, K. Kiran Kumar, and Bramah Hazela. "Scada energy management system under the distributed decimal of service attack using verification techniques by IIoT." In *2023 International Conference on Artificial Intelligence and Knowledge Discovery in Concurrent Engineering (ICECONF)*, pp. 1–4. IEEE, 2023.
10. Patel, Mohit, Harsh Amin, Geetesh Pandey, and Ganesh Wadmare. "Enhancing disaster response training through immersive AR/VR simulations." In *2023 6th International Conference on Advances in Science and Technology (ICAST)*, pp. 69–74. IEEE, 2023.
11. Gundran, Carlos Primero D., et al. "Simulation training needs assessment for disaster preparedness and disaster response among selected agencies in National Capital Region, Philippines." *International Journal of Disaster Risk Reduction* 94 (2023): 103824.
12. Rathore, P. S., S. Ahuja, S. R. Burri, A. Khunteta, A. Baliyan, & A. Kumar. (2024). *Deep learning techniques for automation and industrial applications*. John Wiley & Sons, Inc.; Scrivener Publishing LLC.
13. Tatsuno, Sheridan. "Virtual reality for disaster management and recovery." In Deog-Seong Oh, Fred Young Phillips, and Avvari V Mohan (eds) *SMART CITY 2.0: Strategies and Innovations for City Development*. 2023. 349–356.
14. Bugli, Dante, et al. "Training the public health emergency response workforce: a mixed-methods approach to evaluating the virtual reality modality." *BMJ Open* 13.5 (2023): e063527.
15. Kao, Chia-Lung, et al. "The development of new remote technologies in disaster medicine education: a scoping review." *Frontiers in Public Health* 11 (2023): 1029558.
16. Luo, Yuan, Jun Zhu, Ping Pang, Xianjue Xu, and Yu Qing. "Improving Well Control Response Ability via Virtual Reality Technology." In *Abu Dhabi International Petroleum Exhibition and Conference*, p. D011S014R002. SPE, 2024.
17. Baraldo, Matteo, and Paola Di Giuseppantonio Di Franco. "Place-centred emerging technologies for disaster management: a scoping review." *International Journal of Disaster Risk Reduction* 112 (2024): 104782.
18. De Fino, Mariella, et al. "Boosting urban community resilience to multi-hazard scenarios in open spaces: a virtual reality–serious game training prototype for heat wave protection and earthquake response." *Sustainable Cities and Society* 99 (2023): 104847.
19. Kang, Hosan, et al. "Integrated augmented and virtual reality technologies for realistic fire drill training." *IEEE Computer Graphics and Applications* 44 (2023): 89–99.
20. Heldring, Sara, et al. "Using high-fidelity virtual reality for mass-casualty incident training by first responders–a systematic review of the literature." *Prehospital and Disaster Medicine* 39 (2024): 1–12.
21. Balahadia, F., and J. Sayaman. "Development and evaluation of TYFIREQUAKE: a virtual reality simulation for disaster preparedness of children." *International Journal of Computer Science* 7 (2023): 1385–1418.

22. Chen, Shih-Yeh, and Wei-Che Chien. "Immersive virtual reality serious games with DL-assisted learning in high-rise fire evacuation on fire safety training and research." *Frontiers in Psychology* 13 (2022): 786314.
23. Radhika, Kiran, Bir Kaur, and Salil Bharany. "10 Augmented Reality and Virtual Reality in disaster management systems: A review." *Handbook of Augmented and Virtual Reality* 1 (2023): 155.
24. Hosseini, Mohsen Masoumian, Seyedeh Toktam Masoumian Hosseini, and Karim Qayumi. "A guide to opportunities and challenges of developing a virtual reality simulation for disaster medicine courses: a letter to editor." *Archives of Academic Emergency Medicine* 12.1 (2024).
25. Alene, Gebray H., et al. "Virtual reality visualization of geophysical flows: a framework." *Environmental Modelling & Software* 177 (2024): 106063.

CHAPTER 8

IoT-Enabled Augmented Reality for Real-Time Equipment Diagnosis

Ravi Kumar Vankayalapati, Tulasi Naga Subhash Polineni, Sk Hasane Ahammad, Chandrashekar Pandugula, and R. Senthamil Selvan

8.1 INTRODUCTION

Developments in the Internet of Things (IoT) and augmented reality (AR) technologies greatly aid in the development of novel solutions with distinctive features for user interaction [1]. Applications may benefit from the new features that AR and IoT may provide, enabling them to support complex use situations and successfully handle the difficulties and demands for flawless user experiences [2]. Promoting users' physical activity has long been necessary in the healthcare and assisted living sectors since it significantly decreases due to current living conditions [3–5]. Interventions and rewards for regularly adhering to a care plan are also necessary in many situations [6].

AR technology allows users to see virtual, computer-generated information superimposed on top of their actual, physical surroundings in real time. These days, AR solutions are par for the course in the gaming business, and many game situations encourage players to do more exercise [7]. Exergames are video games that force players to engage in physical activity they don't usually engage in [8–10]. Gamification techniques are needed to make these kinds of serious games work, and the different game goals

DOI: 10.1201/9781003564904-8

force players to face both mental and physical difficulties that will help them improve their health and way of life, mostly over the medium to long term. Improving physical activity usually involves using, setting up, and customizing pricey gear like gaming consoless, external components, sensors, cameras, and more [11–14]. The goal is to provide a working model for serious exergame development that may aid in the evaluation of user health and risk identification while encouraging healthy lifestyle choices. To assure ease of use, compatibility with other platforms, integration with emerging technologies, and cost-effectiveness, the entire system must adhere to a modular architecture and utilize commercially available technology. By using specially designed IoT technologies, the suggested AR game creation platform includes tools for forward-thinking interaction and accurate monitoring of users' activity and vital signs. A mobile framework ready for augmented reality is one of the prototype's main parts. Another is an app for IoT wearables that track user activity and biological signals. Last but not least, there is a web application endpoint-based cloud architecture that enables remote setup and viewing of outcomes by healthcare experts. The Internet of Things is used to monitor physiological signals and motion during gameplay, while AR development principles are employed to enhance immersion.

To provide gameplay independent of a fixed location, ease of use, wireless configuration, and fitness tracking, gaming and AR exergames in commercial devices and on various hardware systems require a combination of approaches and technologies that are not currently available in the state of research [15]. Using the state-of-the-art capabilities of cloud systems, data integration, IoT, and AR for smartphones, this study suggests a solution that successfully meets the aforementioned requirements [16–19]. The suggested platform for exergame development's main benefit is that no extra equipment is needed to play the game or do different tasks. This means that there are no extra costs or restrictions on where the game can be played because of equipment needs. A lot of smart devices can handle it, which makes it easy to access and use. Users, or players, can use AR's advanced interactive features to keep track of their health measures (like heartbeat, step count, and hand tremors) while they play and save the results. A healthcare professional may alter and modify the game elements based on the user's condition along with the treatment plan, after looking at the activities and biological signal data from the watched game events [20]. When showing in-game data in real time, the user interface makes things easy for everyone. The beneficial influence on users' health and physical activity is shown by this example, which also highlights the advantages of implementing augmented reality smartphone exercise games and remote tracking in healthcare use cases. The game's findings demonstrate that players of all ages have fun while playing, which increases their activity level in a fun and creative manner and keeps their brains and bodies working.

The remainder of the chapter is organized as follows: In Section 8.2, the construction, system design, and execution of the prototype are described, together with an analysis of the relevant research on augmented reality, exercising, and IoT for healthcare and supported living situations. Section 8.3 presents performance, medical outcomes, and real-time gaming situations extracted from the programme under real-time settings. In addition to outlining potential future developments for the work, it has been compared to similar applications and technologies in Section 8.4.

8.2 MATERIALS AND METHODS

8.2.1 Architecture of the System

AR is used to show items in the user's home surroundings and encourage them to engage with them. This approach functions as a type of interactive serious gaming. Simultaneously, personal user data is recorded so that they can be watched from configures the game's settings and scenarios. A healthcare worker can use this tool to keep an eye on the users' progress, adjust the game's settings, and review the results of both the game outcomes and the health data. Figure 8.1 gives an overview of the method.

8.2.1.1 Framework for the Development of Augmented Reality Games [Applications for Smart Phones]

This mobile app incorporates the main features of the game framework. When launched, a camera window opens up to display the user's surroundings, and the game overlays different tasks on their screen. AR is used to project interactive options and activities onto real-world surfaces. The player is required to move about and interact with virtual objects as part of predetermined game activities. The process of displaying and selecting replies is one of the AR features that was developed using the Google ARCore platform. Other AR libraries may accomplish comparable outcomes; however, this framework was chosen because of its smooth interface with the Android environment. Similar outcomes are shown by Apple's ARKit, a smartphone that makes use of AR components. However, creating ARKit needs not only Apple testing equipment but also Apple computer

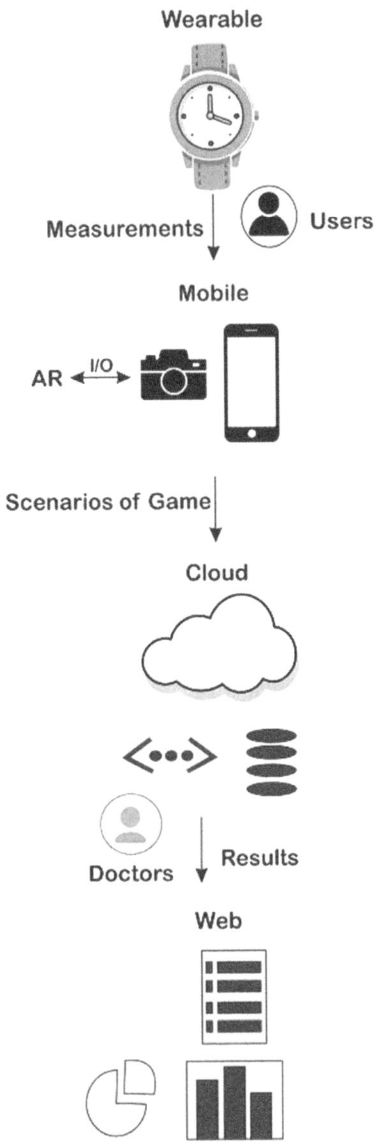

FIGURE 8.1 An overview of the method.

hardware and unique licensing, which restricts developer flexibility. By launching a web browser window, users of mobile devices may access the lightweight AR.js library for the web. Although ARCore and ARKit, based on the platform, supply their essential AR components upon accessing the native device level, Babylon.js and AR libraries support mobile devices.

The user has the option to choose the types and levels of game missions before starting the game, or a healthcare professional may pre-configure them in the situation of a tailored treatment plan using the online application. The smartphone app's duties extend beyond just playing the game to include collecting and analyzing data from the system's compatible sensors. Utilizing the raw data collected by the accelerometer detectors, these measures mostly pertain to the user's hand shaking and movement. Following each successful or failed test, a score is computed in addition to the recorded health metrics. The healthcare professional's web app receives these findings using cloud computing.

8.2.1.2 Applications for Smartwatches

Integration with tools for exercise tracking and biological signal readings is a key part of the system. A smartwatch app can be downloaded and incorporated into a gadget that is paired to the smartphone to make the features work. This automatically opens the app if a game session begins, and while the game is going on Bluetooth technology lets the tracker and mobile apps interact with each other continuously. The smartwatch tracks the wearer's heart rate, moves, and steps, sending the information to a mobile app while showing the results on the watch's face in real time.

8.2.1.3 Services in the Cloud and Web-Based Programmes

The web app is an organizational hub where healthcare supervisors personalize games and monitor what their users are doing. A user's place in the game's leaderboards and their gaming history are both viewable to them. The user's supervisor can access a log of all their gaming sessions and see details such as how long each game lasted, the number of times the user got a question right or wrong, and the total score. Line graphs and pie charts also show health-related statistics like steps, heartbeat, and handshaking. Both the people keeping checks on viewers and the users themselves may benefit from the categorization and evaluation of this data. The supervisor may customize the user tests by setting the content and complexity of the tasks and categories either for all games or for individual users. A cloud platform without servers is used for data sharing among smartphones and web apps. These apps make it easier to set up and launch the platform and game parts. They also improve privacy, adaptability, and scaling, and they make it easier to keep an eye on the system to make sure it runs smoothly. It handles contact among web and mobile apps and stores game settings, results, and measures. It also acts as a bridge between them.

8.2.2 AR Characteristics

The Sceneform library, a three-dimensional architecture that includes a physically dependent renderer designed for mobile devices, is integrated to provide a gamified experience. This makes it simple to create augmented reality applications without the need for Vulkan. Sceneform's API enables ARCore capabilities with Android classes and interfaces. By utilizing the technology of the mobile device and making use of the library's capabilities, ARCore provides users with an augmented reality experience. The library provides an AR fragment, which is a fragment widget that displays the game's user interface. In this section, the camera view is shown with other 3D objects, called anchors, that are created by the AR. A dynamic form like a cube, rectangle, triangle, or the anchor's 3D model may be generated. With the support of the app's plane detection components, the anchors can maintain their positions with ease. These anchors are placed on detected planes, which serve as surfaces inside the environment. The planes serve only for identifying and categorizing surfaces; they are not visible to the camera. Employing AR fragments as its initialization, all of these user interface components are customized in a Sceneform view.

Besides frame update handlers, there are callbacks for changes in the external environment and for finding points and paths. As soon as the session begins, the device logs what the camera observes, figures out what is in front of it, and divides surfaces into groups so that planes can be created. It also keeps track of the locations of all the planes and lets you add, change, or remove planes. It is possible to figure out the distance that exists between two random planes or between a plane and the device. These factors are used during game runtimes to make sure users have a smooth experience and make the game features feel like they belong in the real world.

8.2.3 Platform for Gaming

The suggested solution's prototype incorporates a framework for creating serious augmented reality games, tasks, and obstacles that make use of pre-existing game characteristics and components. Every game incorporates a variety of question types and difficulty levels into its series. To make the gamification concept a reality for users, various metrics and settings are used for each level. Healthcare providers may use the web interface to configure the game's overall setup, which includes all operating factors, levels, and challenges. Notably, these settings may be customized for each user and adjusted while the simulation is running. This allows for a more tailored simulation that operates according to the needs of the care plan and the unique use situation. Professionals can assess many aspects of users' physical and mental health while also successfully encouraging them to engage in certain activities within the framework of a customized care plan by using the game's metrics and settings. The following categories serve as the foundation for the collection of queries that will be asked during a session:

- The user is prompted with a text question, and the responses are shown in the AR section. For situations dependent on knowledge, the responses may take the form of numbers, like the output of a mathematical equation, or they might take the form of language.
- The researcher provides the user with a scenario that has three items such as animals, objects, or balls and asks them to choose the proper animal.
- Three boxes are shown around the person in this type of question. Individuals must walk through these boxes to find the answers that are concealed inside them.
- The user is required to arrange unsorted responses in ascending order according to their links with one another. Typically, the format of this inquiry involves categorizing numbers, months, days of the week, and so on.

8.2.4 Process of Implementation

The system is split into three applications. Each application is made up of a group of different parts that work together to do the task it needs to do. As part of the general system design, one of the major goals is to meet the needs for flexibility and scalability for the expansion of the system in future. As a result, the platform's parts are made to be as simple as possible, with precise interfaces and abstraction sections, while still keeping speed and efficiency high. It is easier for third-party services to work with this app because of the design tools and languages that were used after they were selected. This also makes it possible to connect to other apps in the future.

Two system elements that operate within the framework of the smartphone programme are the menu controller and the game controller. The step tracker and heart rate sensor of wearable apps handle recording and transmitting information to the mobile device. Examples of web apps involve the web-based result manager, which shows the outcomes of previous gaming events, and the online game supervisor, which configures the game's settings. Controllers for synchronization, authentication, and storage make up the cloud platform component. Storage controllers are in charge of keeping track of health information, game situations, and game outcomes, while controllers for authentication and synchronization manage user login statuses and data synchronization as needed.

Applications for wearables and mobile devices are created using the Android activity framework. Sensor readings are handled by a single activity in the smartwatch software, which also shows the data on the display and transmits these to the phone application. In contrast, the mobile application has several functions that correlate to the game controller, results manager, and menu manager. There is just one page in the web application. Cloud services from Firebase serve as the foundation for the backend operations. The database facilitates the synchronization and storage of all system information in addition to implementing the link between the online and mobile applications.

A mobile app's menu manager and game controller are in charge of the app's overall flow and communication with other apps. The modules dedicated to managing results and games make up the menu manager. In addition to storing the game results in the cloud for remote access via the web app, the results manager displays this data as grids, graphs, and tables. If a game is ready to begin, the game manager notifies the controller and specifies the game's level and category. These modules make up the game controller component: measurements, ARCore, answer validator, and session. A measurements processor measures tremors, steps, and smartwatch app connection. The ARCore controller offers modelled outputs to the game controller component by manipulating the ARCore and Sceneform libraries. The session controller controls game operations, including receiving the start command, acquiring assets, setting up the ARCore controller, reading measurements, displaying visuals, and managing user interactions.

Sensors on the smartwatch connect to the application, which then send the data to the mobile app through Bluetooth. For technical reasons, the built-in Wear OS API makes it possible to read the sensors and connect to the phone. The processes of the web interface are implemented by the web application components. The supervisor is first presented with the data that the online results manager has retrieved from the cloud storage of the smartphone results manager component. This component also handles the tasks of establishing the game's settings, types, questions, and levels. The results manager activities allow users to examine their performance, points, progress, scores, and other metrics. It is also possible for users to share the findings with their family, friends, or medical professionals.

8.3 RESULTS

8.3.1 System Operation

The game session starts when the menu manager establishes the desired difficulty level and quest type selections in addition to providing the app's basic navigation. To start the session in the app's user interface, the game controller receives this setting and displays the augmented reality action. The system loads the necessary questions and any necessary assets into the memory, depending on the type of mission. After powering up and pairing with the wristwatch app, the measurement controller initializes and prepares the system. Additionally, it sets up the phone's accelerometer and step counter sensors, which will be used if the watch's sensors are unavailable so that it can identify when the user's hands are shaking. Each quest's unique difficulty is iterated through the game. In this setup, the user sees a challenge (or question) written in text at the top of the display, and the augmented reality fragment displays the solutions. A plane is located in the user's immediate vicinity, and each response is shown as an anchor on that plane.

Based on experiments conducted in actual user contexts (e.g., kitchens, living rooms, workplaces, and gardens), we developed an anchor placement algorithm to prevent anchor conflicts. The procedure is conducted for each question as shown in Figure 8.2. As the augmented reality session is established and plane detection begins, a list including the question's responses and associated data (labels, assets, etc.) is saved in the system memory. The method begins by selecting a random plane from the observed options as a potential location for each response. The following

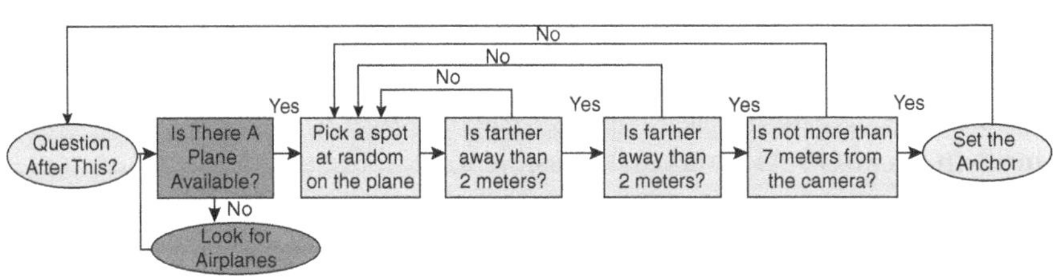

FIGURE 8.2 The procedure is conducted for each question.

criteria are then used to determine whether this site is suitable: the distance from the camera must be more than 2 meters, but less than 7 meters, and the site must be at least 2 meters away from the closest anchor. When these conditions are satisfied, the answer's anchor is set and the related 3D model is safely displayed.

The user's response is saved when they touch on it, and the iteration continues with the following question. Data collected during the session is saved together with the question's outcome. Among these measures are:

- Time required: how long it took the user to discover, capture, reject, or accept the response.
- Missed hits: when you try to capture an answer but fail. When a user ends a session before it has finished, it is considered an incomplete session.
- Steps: the total number of steps tracked by the phone's device.
- Heart rate: the whole sequence of heart rates as recorded by the watch, with minimum, maximum, and average values shown.

Using the phone's accelerometer sensor, we can identify and categorize shaking hands in a waveform style or according to predefined categories depending on the accelerations we observe.

Using the AR fragment's frame update listener, frame rate (FPS) is calculated and exported as min/max/average, which helps with battery consumption. Additionally, the system tracks the percentage change in the current battery's capacity to measure battery drain.

8.3.2 Gameplay

The game shows heart rate, stride, and tremor in real time via augmented reality. The AR game session starts when the user chooses questions, levels, and types (which may be predefined by their doctor). Moving about the environment to grab virtual objects on the screen is the goal of the game. AR item categories depend on the game mission question type. We supported four-game quests. The smartphone used was a Huawei P20 Lite-ANE LX1 (2.36 GHz, 4 GB RAM, 16 MP Camera). Questions of type (a) require the user to identify and touch a 3D model that is shown as the focus of the quest. Responses that are given in free text are shown in (b). Box-type inquiries (type (c)) need the user to touch the box to disclose the potential response. Lastly, the user must choose the solutions that are shown in a certain sequence in type (d). The fact that the player has to move about to get the answers and advance in the game is a benefit of the gameplay. The user's general interests may be used to determine the context of the questions.

8.3.3 Web Applications and Cloud Platforms

The web application, which serves as the platform endpoints for medical practitioners, and the cloud platform, which stores the game scenarios and outcomes, are the main components of the system. The primary features of the web application are shown in Figures 8.3–8.5. Results and rankings are the main foci of the programme, which relies on a scoring system that categorizes users' outcomes. There are three levels proposed in the game scenario prototype: silver, gold, diamond, and challenger. The response screen shows the heart rate and shaking as line and pie charts, respectively. The dashboard shows the remaining metrics.

8.3.4 Performance of the System

An AR exergame that doesn't need any additional hardware is demonstrated in the created prototype smartphone app. Ten tests of the prototype were conducted on four devices—the Huawei P20 Lite, TCL 20 5G, Galaxy A20, and Galaxy A7 2018—for each kind of inquiry. The above data reflect the typical outcomes of ten sessions of each type's performance. There are ten missions in a single session. The percentage of power left in the battery at the beginning and end of each session is used to determine the amount of battery power that is used. All tests are included in the total frame rate.

There are no high-definition graphics or multi-edge polygons, therefore the findings suggest that the choice of box-type questions leads to better playability. The rendering of 3D models (assets) makes object questions the most resource-intensive. Tasks involving text or sorting often include model queries derived from Android UI view elements (TextView, ImageView) may execute more smoothly than object inquiries, but not box questions. The reduced sizes of edges, polygons, colours, and surfaces in Android UI view components provide improved performances compared

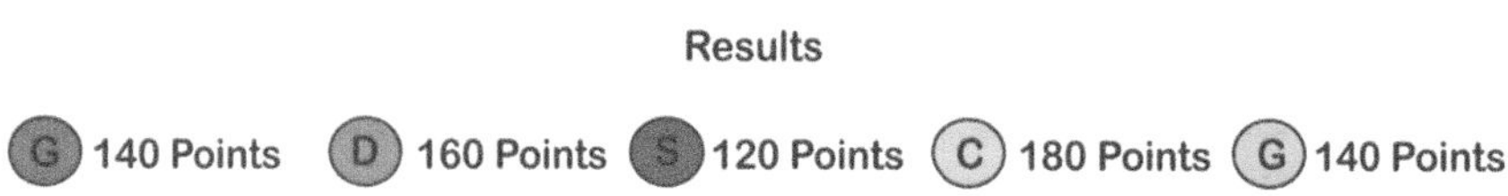

FIGURE 8.3 Dashboard for a web app.

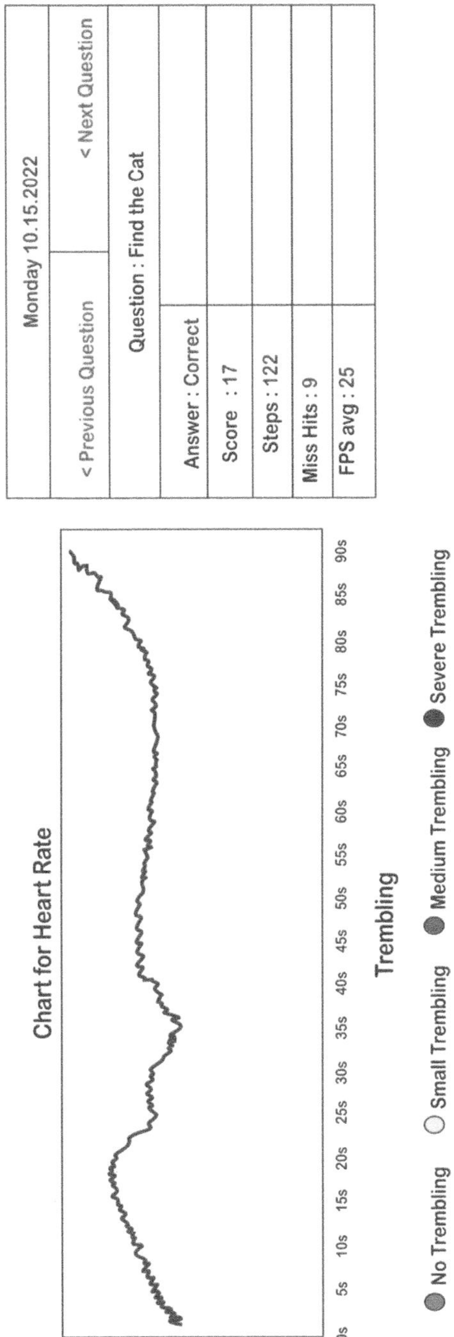

FIGURE 8.4 Score and a graph of heart rate.

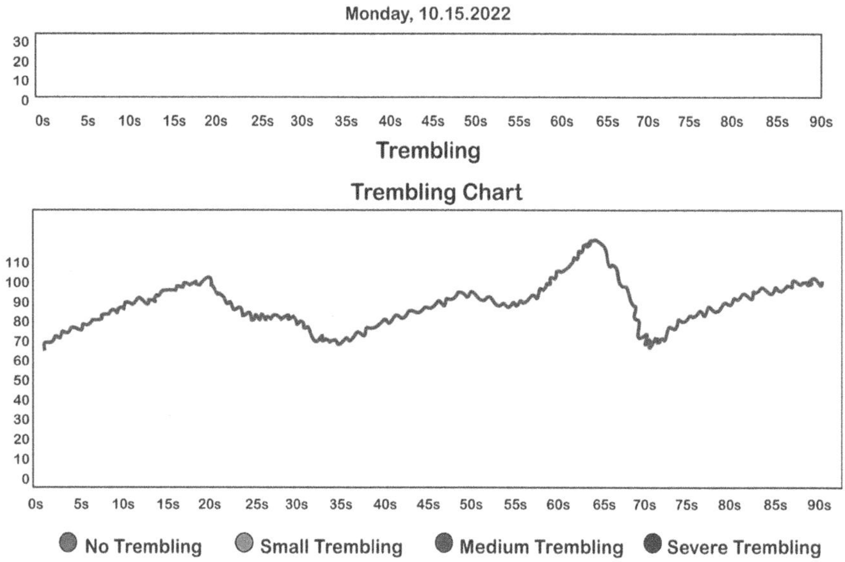

FIGURE 8.5 Chart and picture for trembling.

to 3D models. As long as the frame rate indicator is around 30, the game is enjoyable and no frame dips can be immediately seen, regardless of the variances between the average FPS readings of each question type.

8.3.5 Limitations of the System

The gameplay is unaffected by the many elements that influence the game's performance. There may be screen frame drops if the session lasts longer than intended, depending on the mobile device type, illumination, and display layout. Optimizations for performance and ideas for gameplay are offered to fix this issue:

- Make sure that additional planes aren't detected after all the answers are submitted;
- Make it so that you may only choose up to four answers to each question;
- Recommend playing the game in a bright, spacious area (like a living room or patio).

Additionally, this early version is only compatible with Android smartphones that have Google service installed, but there are plans to integrate it for iOS soon.

8.3.6 Analyzing Games

In addition to the performance study, we also evaluated the fundamental gamification features. To be more precise:

- Fifteen users in their forties and fifties and eighteen users in their thirties made up the test population.
- A smartwatch was used to monitor the steps and heart rate.
- The device's accelerometer was used to determine the vibration, which was then ranked from 1 to 4. Ten sessions of each question type's findings are provided. Users in the 20–40 age group have their average medical metrics, whereas users in the 40–60 age group have the same metrics to each other.

The players are rather active when they are playing the game, maintaining a decent speed and an average heart rate, according to the results. When looking at parameters like game time, steps, and trembling, the findings suggest that the 40–60 age group marginally outperformed the other group, although the heart rate averages went in the other direction.

8.3.7 Technology Evaluation

Building an augmented reality gamification platform and creating a proof of concept for using AR and IoT in the healthcare sector were the primary goals of this project. Consequently, the system's usability and general architecture were the primary foci of the examination. A technological acceptability questionnaire was created and sent out to the aforementioned user groups to assess the system's usefulness. The survey asked participants to rate the following aspects of the product: its perceived utility, simplicity of use, and intention to use it.

Here are the possible responses: –3 (Completely disagree), –2 (Disagree), –1 (Slightly disagree), 0 (Not at all), 1 (Somewhat agree), 2 (Agree), 3 (Strongly agree) (Figure 8.6).

The findings show that users had nothing but praise for the augmented reality gaming system and had nothing but great things to say about the

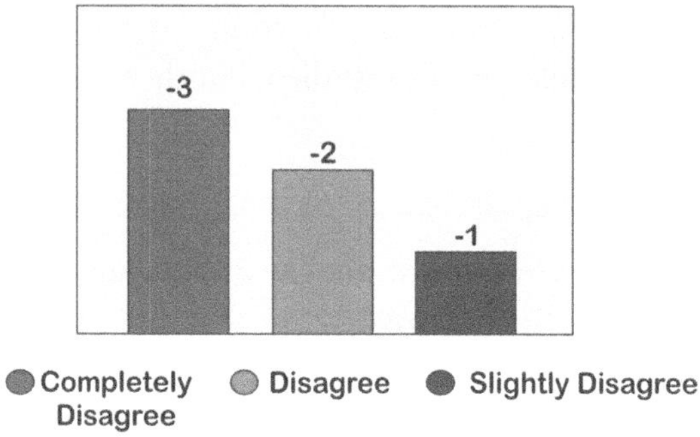

FIGURE 8.6 Bar chart for possible responses.

effect it had on their health. The system's usefulness, particularly in cramped quarters and other complex settings, can need some work.

8.4 DISCUSSION AND CONCLUSION

Users and healthcare providers alike will reap the advantages of the suggested solution's integrated and flexible environment, cutting-edge technology, and tools for system configuration and monitoring. In contrast to previous health-focused serious games, this augmented reality prototype monitors crucial elements of players' physical and mental health without requiring costly and supplementary hardware like gaming consoles, additional modules, cameras, displays, and so on.

The portability and convenience of being able to conduct augmented reality sessions from the comfort of one's own home are other advantages of the smartphone app. This outcome is made possible by a software setup and technique that continuously accounts for the state of the actual world and the associated physical constraints. Anyone, including those without much technical knowledge, may utilize this hybrid experience with ease because of the user-friendly and accessible design.

Additionally, a wearable device is used to track health data, promote the quantified self approach, and provide a comprehensive clinical overview of users' physical status during gameplay. Healthcare serious game concepts that combine augmented reality with the Internet of Things are unusual. The proposed system stands out due to its IoT sensor integration and its ready-to-use augmented reality game development environment. In this way, patients and doctors may work together to develop individualized treatment programmes, increase exercise, and holistically improve health.

The game's engaging nature and gaming experience encourages players, together with its cutting-edge technology. Its diverse gaming scenarios and numerous features keep users interested, reducing the likelihood of obsolescence. The fact that healthcare experts are involved in designing the game, creating scenarios, and setting challenges motivates users to utilize the system because they feel it is suited to their needs. The system motivates users to exercise and improve their mental health through well-designed gaming challenges. The mobile and online applications' score and ranking systems make the game more competitive and fun. The online application displays detailed analytics and metrics using charts and pie graphs. Another benefit is that healthcare professionals actively participate in the system, evaluate game outcomes, and configure operational and gaming settings. The online tool lets healthcare professionals watch and provide feedback to users while exercising. The online application's ability to set up game sessions allows professionals to configure game conditions, replay games, and track user physical progress in addition to outcomes tracking. In addition to exercise encouragement, this system may enhance user well-being by obtaining health data that can identify an illness. For example, using the device's accelerometer sensor, hand tremor raw data may be used to diagnose muscular or neurological disorders.

This work's key novel contributions are not yet accessible as a single offering. The suggested solution integrates one-of-a-kind gamification features and technologies with the Internet of Things and augmented reality in healthcare, resulting in a state-of-the-art development platform that healthcare providers may use to build novel, interactive environments for patient monitoring and interaction.

The solution's single offering literature evaluation and capacity comparison demonstrate its potential to help develop novel therapies as part of a customized care plan. Healthcare professionals may alter system parameters and create new game conditions in the recommended advanced remote monitoring system. The proof-of-concept prototype shows the platforms' synergy and commercial hardware capabilities. This platform proposes a physical activity exergame prototype that monitors user measurements, offers physicians real-time health data, and enables them to pre-define and remotely operate the game using IoT, AR, cloud, and online technologies. The hardware-agnostic software may operate on commercially available, pre-owned devices, cutting ownership expenses. It may increase user knowledge and provide a novel way to improve quantified self-assisted living well-being.

Future developments will add more features to provide healthcare practitioners with a more complete picture of users' health and cognition. Integrating affective computing frameworks to analyze users' emotions is one example. Further testing will evaluate whether other AR and conventional computer vision engines can handle similar use scenarios. Better gameplay will enable more sophisticated real-world interactions, which will be used to create more complicated game challenges and situations. Users' care plans will determine obstacles, and rules for dynamic game parameter modifications depending on the care plan and observed outcomes will be established in partnership with healthcare experts. This plugin will combine quantified-self recommendation implementations. For improved user experience and more thrilling gameplay, multi-user activities will be enabled locally and remotely.

REFERENCES

1. Liu, Changchun, et al. "Probing an intelligent predictive maintenance approach with deep learning and augmented reality for machine tools in IoT-enabled manufacturing." *Robotics and Computer-Integrated Manufacturing* 77 (2022): 102357.
2. Zhang, Zixuan, et al. "Artificial intelligence-enabled sensing technologies in the 5G/internet of things era: from virtual reality/augmented reality to the digital twin." *Advanced Intelligent Systems* 4.7 (2022): 2100228.
3. Chen, Po-Hsuan Cameron, et al. "An augmented reality microscope with real-time artificial intelligence integration for cancer diagnosis." *Nature Medicine* 25.9 (2019): 1453–1457.
4. Wang, Shaohan, Sakib Ashraf Zargar, and Fuh-Gwo Yuan. "Augmented reality for enhanced visual inspection through knowledge-based deep learning." *Structural Health Monitoring* 20.1 (2021): 426–442.
5. Stark, Erich, et al. "Using augmented reality and internet of things for control and monitoring of mechatronic devices." *Electronics* 9.8 (2020): 1272.
6. Manda JK. Augmented Reality (AR) Applications in Telecom Maintenance: Utilizing AR Technologies for Remote Maintenance and Troubleshooting in Telecom Infrastructure. Available at SSRN 5136767. 2023 Aug 23.
7. Rajulu, G. Govinda, M. Jamuna Rani, D. Deepa, Udit Mamodiya, Radhika G. Deshmukh, and T. Rajasanthosh Kumar. "Cloud-Computed Solar Tracking System." *Computer Communication, Networking and IoT* 2 (2021): 75.
8. Vogt, Sebastian. *Real-Time Augmented Reality for Image-Guided Interventions.* Dissertation. Friedrich-Alexander-Universität Erlangen-Nürnberg (FAU), 2009.
9. Dhotre, Virendrakumar Anna, et al. "Big data analytics using MapReduce for the education system." *Linguistica Antverpiensia* (2021): 3130–3138.
10. Lee, Sanghoon, and Ömer Akin. "Augmented reality-based computational fieldwork support for equipment operations and maintenance." *Automation in Construction* 20.4 (2011): 338–352.
11. Rai, Rahul, et al. "Machine learning in manufacturing and industry 4.0 applications." *International Journal of Production Research* 59.16 (2021): 4773–4778.

12. BramahHazela, J. Hymavathi, T. Rajasanthosh Kumar, S. Kavitha, D. Deepa, Sachin Lalar, and Prabakaran Karunakaran. "Machine Learning: Supervised Algorithms to Determine the Defect in High-Precision Foundry Operation." *Journal of Nanomaterials* 2022.1 (2022): 1732441.
13. Angrisani, Leopoldo, et al. "A wearable brain-computer interface instrument for augmented reality-based inspection in industry 4.0." *IEEE Transactions on Instrumentation and Measurement* 69.4 (2019): 1530–1539.
14. Tai, Yonghang, et al. "Trustworthy and intelligent COVID-19 diagnostic iomt through xr and deep-learning-based clinic data access." *IEEE Internet of Things Journal* 8.21 (2021): 15965–15976.
15. Douglas, David B., et al. "Augmented reality: advances in diagnostic imaging." *Multimodal Technologies and Interaction* 1.4 (2017): 29.
16. Bai, Li, et al. "Chinese experts' consensus on the Internet of Things-aided diagnosis and treatment of coronavirus disease 2019 (COVID-19)." *Clinical eHealth* 3 (2020): 7–15.
17. Erkoyuncu, John Ahmet, et al. "Improving the efficiency of industrial maintenance with context-aware adaptive authoring in augmented reality." *CIRP Annals* 66.1 (2017): 465–468.
18. Chen, Yi-Jao, Yong-Shan Lai, and Yen-Han Lin. "BIM-based augmented reality inspection and maintenance of fire safety equipment." *Automation in Construction* 110 (2020): 103041.
19. Sadhu, Ayan, et al. "A review of data management and visualization techniques for structural health monitoring using BIM and virtual or augmented reality." *Journal of Structural Engineering* 149.1 (2023): 03122006.
20. Ma, Marco King In, et al. "Virtual reality and augmented reality—emerging screening and diagnostic techniques in ophthalmology: a systematic review." *Survey of Ophthalmology* 67.5 (2022): 1516–1530.

CHAPTER 9

AR/VR-Based Disaster Simulation for Community Resilience Training

Charanjeet Singh, Guna Sekhar Sajja, K. Suresh Kumar, Pramoda Patro, and M. Clement Joe Anand

9.1 INTRODUCTION

As IoT technology advances, industrial equipment intelligence has increased, leading to increasingly complex structures. Meanwhile, due to the complex and unpredictable operating circumstances and harsh environments, industrial equipment systems are more prone to performance degradation and failure rates. Failures in major equipment systems may create accidents that result in severe economic losses and even fatalities. To avoid such occurrences, significant human and financial resources are required to enhance equipment security and stability. According to the research, equipment maintenance costs in manufacturing contribute to the overall production costs. Early and accurate prediction of system remaining usable life (RUL) is crucial to prevent major mishaps, particularly in the beginning stages of equipment system deterioration. Effective maintenance is crucial for ensuring the safe and reliable functioning of IoT-based industrial systems.

Prognostics and Health Management (PHM) technology is crucial to assess contemporary mechanical devices. A suitable PHM system can

DOI: 10.1201/9781003564904-9

accurately monitor mechanical equipment and suggest an efficient maintenance plan. Additionally, it predicts system reliability and RUL to avoid faultsaintainPHM strategies, and improve manufacturing efficiency. Deep learning excels at fitting non-linear functions and capturing latent functional relationships in time series data. In recent years, deep learning–based algorithms have been a popular focus in PHM research.

For RUL prediction, fault characteristics have been retrieved using several methods. In deep belief networks (DBNs) for bevel gear RUL prediction, six vibrating state indicators such as Root Mean Square (RMS) and modulation of frequencies are used as health pointers. Deep neural networks use spectral data. The ERBM estimates the RUL of rolling bearings using time and frequency domain data. Information about time, frequency, and time-frequency was retrieved from vibration data using a multimodal deep classification of support for the vector's technique. The Gaussian-Bernoulli algorithms also have identified gear faults in each DBM feature set. An LSTM-based feature fusion approach for RUL prediction combines many feature data to build a health factor with high prediction accuracy. A deep feature of the learning approach uses frequency-time representation and a multi-scale convolutional neural network (CNN) to reliably forecast the remaining life. Additionally, correlation analysis has been used to extract time-varying vibration signal properties using a three-layer FNN. Finally, the scale was fed the projected time-varying vibration signal properties. The risk model estimates the survival and hazard rates of a bearing, predicting its RUL. The experiment demonstrated the rationality and dependability of the RUL prediction approach. A one-dimensional CNN was used to suggest a defect diagnostic approach for the power transformers. This allows the suggested strategy to withstand uncertainty and attain a more robust system.

1. Although the following RUL prediction algorithms have strong theoretical outcomes, professional signal processing and domain-specialized skills are needed for many practical applications of machines deteriorating differently. Manual features of learning engineering reduce modelling generality.

   Equipment modelling becomes more challenging under complex operating conditions. Thus, replacing the manual annotation with an automated method that universally pulls valuable properties from complex signals is essential.

2. The current maintenance technique uses printed instructions and human skills. Poor efficiency and frequent mis-operations may occur from maintenance staff failing to adapt to quick equipment updates in the production of systems.

This study suggests a deep learning–based augmented reality-assisted PHM to solve IoT-enabled industrial problems. Primary contributions fall into two categories.

- PSO-CNN–based feature extraction is used to find internal correlations in the big production statistics sets. The RUL forecast uses GRU (gate returning unit) attention. This technique solves the gradient disappearance problem and captures both the short-term and long-term time series connections. GRU and attention mechanisms may provide higher accuracy predictions.
- Augmented reality delivers immersive settings with visual instructions for effective maintenance recommendations. Maintenance workers may also request remote expert help for complicated situations they cannot fix.

In Section 9.2, research on deep learning in RUL, health management, prognostics, and AR-based maintenance is presented. Section 9.3 focuses on building the framework architecture of the solution. In Section 9.4, the framework is put into action with the help of an AR and an RUL prediction model that is enabled by deep learning keeping up with the actual world. In Section 9.5 are the results from an actual workshop that used the Internet of Things to facilitate production. The final section confirms the efficacy of the proposed method and comparative tests are conducted. Section 9.7 provides a summary and predictions.

9.2 SYSTEM ARCHITECTURE

The production of the data module, the RUL forecast module, and the AR-assisted maintenance module make up the framework design for an AR-based PHM system that is powered by deep learning (Figure 9.1). The detailed explanation of each specific component is as follows:

- **Production Data Module**:

  Acquisition of production data from robots, autonomous ground vehicles, and machine tools falls within the preview of this module.

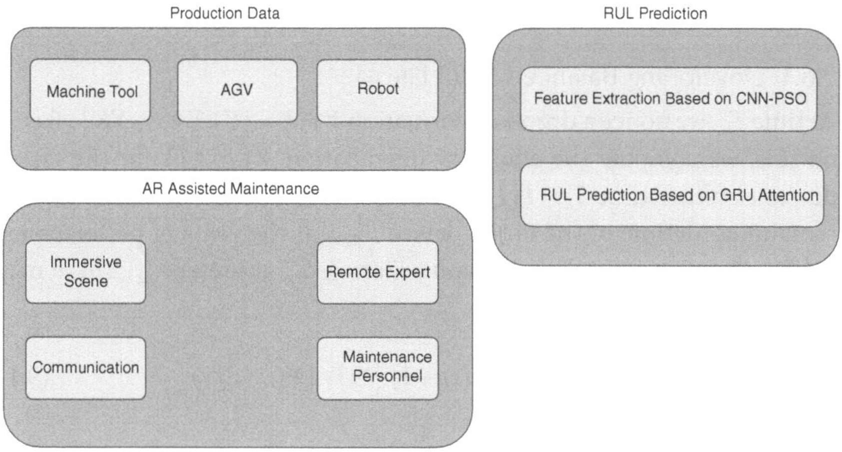

FIGURE 9.1 Schematic view of AR-assisted PHM system.

Data normalization and cleaning may then be used to preprocess the production data. The task of eliminating anomalous data falls to data cleansing. A dimensional expression may be changed into a production of data and a scalar value by using data normalization. Data allows the model to extract important information while avoiding irrelevant information.

- **RUL Forecast Module**:

  A PSO-CNN–based feature extraction approach is suggested for searching the enormous data set for an unidentified connection. Through its convolution and pooling procedures, CNN is tasked with extracting the key elements. Consequently, the CNN-based fault feature extraction algorithm is fine-tuned by leveraging PSO's optimization function to boost feature extraction efficiency. The RUL estimation is achieved using GRU, which depends on the high-efficiency extraction of attributes. By combining GRU with the attention mechanism, researchers can reach a higher accuracy prediction result.

- **AR-Assisted Maintenance Module**:

  AR is used to create a realistic 3D environment maintaining information and instructions to provide high-efficiency servicing support. The WebRTC communication system lets repair workers receive assistance from a remote expert when they are having tough issues that they can't handle on their own. Maintenance workers can connect with the realistic virtual environment and do their jobs effectively with the support of clear, visible instructions.

9.3 FRAMEWORK IMPLEMENTATION

9.3.1 Developing Balance Useful Life

At time T_k, we notice a drop in information $Y1:k=\{Y1,Y2,\ldots,YK\}$. Based on this, we compute the efficiency degradation $Y(T_k+I)$ for the target device at future time $T_k+I\,(I>0)$. Time I may be used to determine the remaining lifetime of the target device T_{REM} if the value of performance $Y(T_k+1)$ first approaches the fault criterion T_f at present t_k. These may be stated in the following way:

$$T_{\text{REM}}=\inf[I:Y(t_k+I_k]\geq T_f\,|\,Y(t_0<T_f) \tag{9.1}$$

The following describes the remaining life probabilities density function for the target device where the random variables are $\mu_{\beta,k}$ and $\sigma_{\beta,k}$ at present T_k:

$$f_{T_{\text{REM}}(I_I|x_{I:K})}\approx\frac{1}{A^*}gT_{\text{REM}}(I_I\,|\,Y_{I:k}) \tag{9.2}$$

$$A^*=\int_0^\infty\frac{1}{A^*}gT_{\text{REM}}(u)du \tag{9.3}$$

Therefore, the numerical integration may be used to characterize the target machine's allocating functions as follows:

$$F_T(t)=P[T\leq t]=\int_0^t f_T(u)du \tag{9.4}$$

9.3.2 Deep Learning–Based RUL Prediction

This section suggests a deep learning–enabled method to increase the RUL prediction model's effectiveness and accuracy. Following is a description of the RUL prediction process utilizing PSO-CNN and GRU–Attention.

- **Data**: Prior to being fed into CNN, the production data undergoes preprocessing and sampling. This allows CNN to more accurately detect the signal.
- **Model for feature extraction**: First, the convolutional layer for the CNN propagation model is used to extract features from the

production data. Next, the feature data's dimension may be decreased via the pooling layer. Finally, the CNN-based fault feature extraction system is modified to increase feature extraction efficiency by using the PSO optimization feature.

- **Model for RUL prediction**: Machine learning algorithms like CNN use GRU to find connections between data. Users will pay more attention to important information because of the attention process. This means that the RUL forecast model will be more accurate.

9.3.2.1 Using PSO-CNN for Fault Feature Extraction

The method for figuring out the layer of convolution is expressed as:

$$x_j^n = F(\sum_{i \in M_j} x_i^{n-1} K_{ij}^n + b_j^n \tag{9.5}$$

The method for figuring out the layer of pooling is represented as:

$$x_j^{n+1} = F(\sum_j x_j^n w_j^{n+1} + b_j^{n+1} \tag{9.6}$$

The result of the output layer is provided as follows:

$$y = f_n\left[\ldots\left(f_2\left(f_1\left(x.w^1\right)w^2\right)\right)\ldots\right]w^n \tag{9.7}$$

The error function is indicated as:

$$Er = \frac{1}{n}\sum_{i=1}^{N}\left(y_{ji}^d - y_{ji}\right)^2 \tag{9.8}$$

The following is the expression for the position and velocity update formulae, respectively:

$$x_i\left(t+1\right) = x_i\left(t\right) + V_i\left(t+1\right) \tag{9.9}$$

$$V_i\left(t+1\right) = \omega V_i\left(t\right) + A_1U_1\left(P_i - x_i\left(t\right)\right) + A_2U_2\left(P_i - x_i\left(t\right)\right) \tag{9.10}$$

Where the constants A_1 and A_2 representacceleration factors and ω denotes the inertia factor. Unintentional numbers produced in (0,1) are represented by U_1 and U_2. In addition, particle I's location in the iteration is denoted by $x_i(t)$, and its velocity in that iteration is denoted by $V_i(t)$.

To employ the PSO to improve CNN settings, follow these steps:

Step 1: Initialize the particle settings.

Step 2: Define the value range for the CNN parameters that need optimization, and utilize that range to change the speed and position of the particles. It is the highest or lowest value in the period that the particles that are outside the value range receive. If a particle moves beyond the defined bounds, it is reset to the nearest limit (either maximum or minimum allowed value).

Step 3: Train CNN on the parameters of each particle and evaluate its accuracy.

Step 4: Use the learnt parameters as the best CNN structure parameters if the training matches the precision standards. If not, go back to step 3.

Step 5: At the IoT-enabled manufacturing workshop, utilize the best settings to examine the CNN and get the feature extraction outcomes of device fault signals.

9.3.2.2 RUL Estimation Using GRU–Attention

The gating signal G_t may be generated by the hidden layer states L_{t-1} and the input X_T, under the influence of σ. A new state S_t is created using this data, which contains all the important input information. A new gating signal GNT can be made by the layer that is hidden state L_t along with the input X_T when σ is applied. It has a pair of elements: r_t and $1-r_t$. The previous time step's hidden state is L_{t-1} and the update status S'_t chooses the next time step's state. From this, the current moment's hidden state L_t can be found and used both to generate the output at the current moment and to serve as input for the next time step. This current hidden state LtL_tLt is then used both to generate the output at the current moment and to serve as input for the next time step. The attention mechanism assigns varying weights to different processing regions to mimic the traits how humans focus attention. This will result in weights being lowered for less essential material and more attention being given to relevant content (distributing big weights). The differential assignment increases processing efficiency and enhances feature extraction quality. Equations (9.11)–(9.13) define the specific calculating procedure.

$$F = \sum_{i=1}^{t} M_i * L_i \tag{9.11}$$

$$M_i = \frac{\exp[Y_i]}{\sum_{k=1}^{t} \exp[e_k]} \tag{9.12}$$

$$Y_i = v_a^T \tanh \tanh(W_i h_i + b_i) \tag{9.13}$$

The weight total of each hidden state in both the input and new hidden states is represented by the vector F. The quantity of information currently held in the concealed state is denoted by Y_i. There are two weight vectors, v_a and W_i, after initializing the network. As the attention mechanism operates, the attention state will be updated by continuously updating the formula's parameters.

9.4 EXPERIMENTAL ENVIRONMENT

Figure 9.2 shows the layout of the typical IoT-enabled machining workplace. Two AGVs, two robots, and four industrial machines make up a typical machining workplace. This allows this workshop to process the

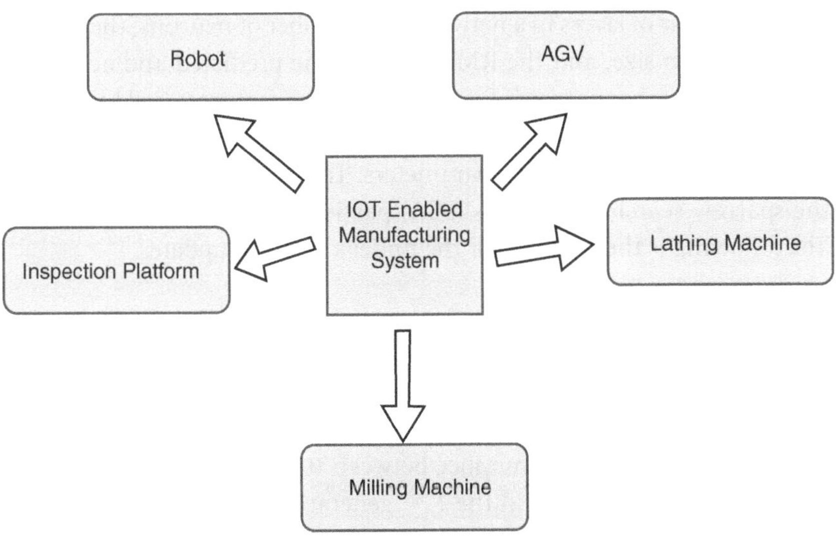

FIGURE 9.2 Block diagram for IOT-based workshop.

boards, flange, and axis. In this workshop, different kinds of sensors like acoustic emission sensors as well as force sensors are employed to collect statistics on production. A normal machine shop can make several unique custom parts, including specialized shaft components, specialized flange items, and customized plate elements.

9.4.1 Defining the Parameters

Table 9.1 displays the outcomes of the GRU layers' adjustments. It demonstrates that a two-layer GRU architecture achieves improved prediction accuracy with less processing time. Because fault features cannot be well analyzed and RUL properties cannot be retrieved with a single GRU layer, the impact is low. Having three GRU layers causes the training period to be excessively lengthy, even if the difference in accuracy is minimal. Overfitting occurs and training time is to be excessive when there are four GRU layers. Consequently, two GRU layers are the ideological zone.

TABLE 9.1 Configuration of the GRU Model's Parameters

GRU Layers	Neurons	Epochs	Batch Size	RMSE	Running Time
1	64	100	128	1.97	528
2	64	100	128	1.04	545
3	64	100	128	1.38	690
4	64	100	128	2.60	857

The number of layers in a network, the number of neurons, the learning rate, the batch size, and the RMSE among the predicted and actual outcomes serve as the sparrow's food (the inputs or features used by the optimization algorithm). Maximizing the RUL forecast model's performance is possible with well-set hyperparameters. The following is a description of the sparrow search algorithm's (SSA) particular computation procedure. The following is the formula for the finder's location update:

$$x_{i,d}\left(t+1\right)=(x_{i,d}\left(t\right).\exp\exp\left[\frac{-i}{\alpha iter_{\max}}\right], \quad A_2<WT\; x_{i,d}\left(t\right)+Q, A_2\geq WT) \tag{9.14}$$

Where α is an arbitrary number between 0 and 1, and $X_I\left(t\right)$ denotes the I^{Th} sparrow's position in the t^{-Th} generations in the d-dimension. At the same time, A_2 is a uniformly random integer between 0 and 1, and

Q is a number drawn at random from the usual normal distribution. The warning threshold is represented by W_T, and intermix represents the total iterations.

The method for updating a follower's place is as follows:

$$x_{i,d}(t+1) = (Q.\exp\exp\left[\frac{xw_d(t) - x_{i,d}(t)}{i^2}\right], i > \frac{N}{2} xb_d(t) \\ + \frac{1}{D}\sum_{d=1}^{D} [rand[-1,1] * [|xb_d(t) - xb_{i,d}(t)|], i \le \frac{N}{2}) \tag{9.15}$$

From each generation, the alter chooses one sparrow at random. That selected sparrow must immediately leave its current position. This is the formula that the alter uses to update its position:

$$x_{i,d}(t+1) = (xb_d(t) + Q * [x_{i,d}(t) - xb_d(t), f_i(t) \\ \neq f_b(t) x_{i,d}(t) + K * \left[\frac{x_{i,d}(t) - xw_d(t)}{|f_i(t) - f_w(t)| + \varepsilon}, f_i(t) = f_b(t)) \right. \tag{9.16}$$

Formula (9.16) shows that the alert sparrow will move to a position near its current location if it is the best individual in the population. If not, it will go in the direction of the best-performing individual. To find high-quality hyperparameter combinations, SSA is used to optimize hyperparameters. Figure 9.3 displays the best fitness update procedure for every generation in the optimization. The precise parameter settings for the suggested RUL prediction model are based on SSA. Overfitting may be successfully avoided by modifying the dropout setting value. This allows for the adjustment of the model's generalization capacity as well as the likelihood that each neuron will be deleted in dropout. The model's generalization of capacity is optimal when the dropout rate is set to 0.5 in this study, which can successfully avoid the overfitting.

9.5 ANALYSIS OF PERFORMANCE AND EXPERIMENTAL RESULTS

9.5.1 RUL Performance Analysis and Forecast Outcome

Figure 9.4(a) and (b) show how the RUL forecast model was trained using the suggested deep learning method. The accuracy and loss metrics were not satisfactory for the initial epochs. The model makes accurate

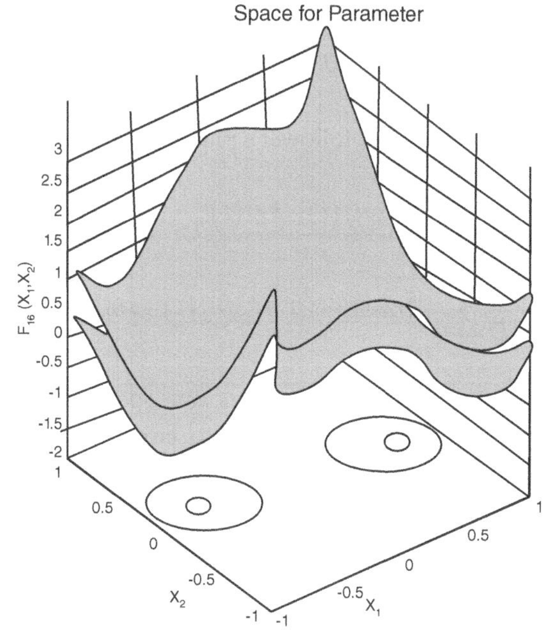

(A) Space for Parameter

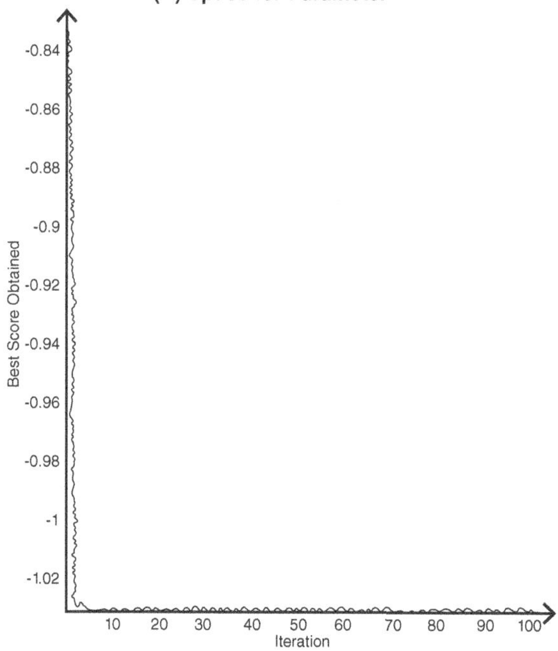

(B) Curve of Iterative

FIGURE 9.3 SSA-based optimization's ideal fitness update. (a) Space for parameter and (b) curve of iterative.

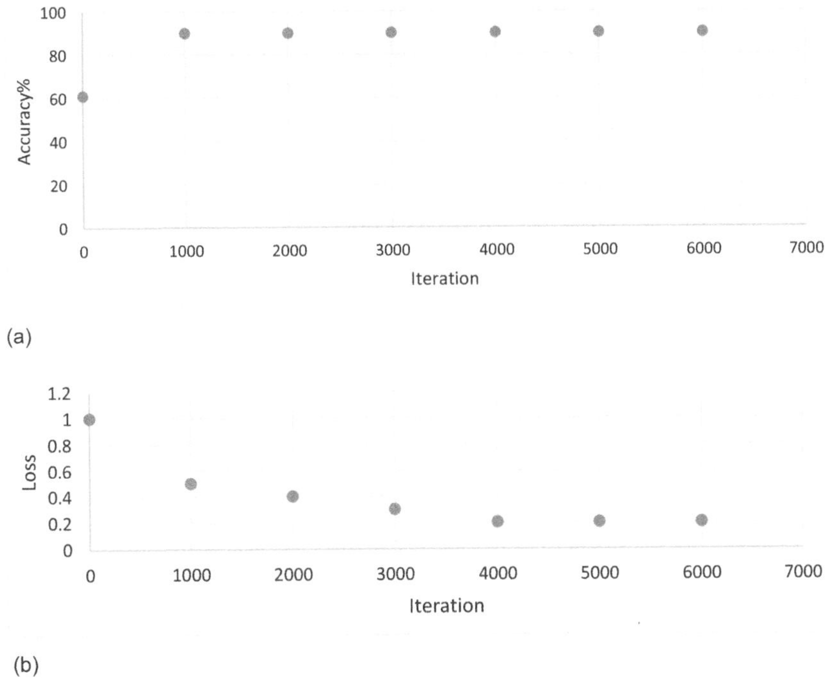

FIGURE 9.4 (a) and (b) RUL prediction model's training procedure.

predictions after being trained for 100 iterations, which is what the training method shows. Finally, 97.64% of the validations are correct.

The results of the RUL prediction using the suggested method are shown in Figure 9.5. In Figure 9.5, the machine tool's RUL prediction result is shown, with the line representing the actual value. This

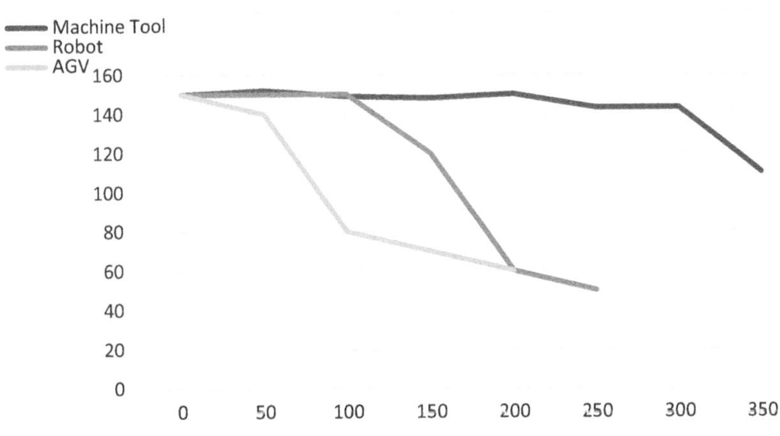

FIGURE 9.5 Predicted RUL value of machine tool, robot, and AGV.

demonstrates that the proposed prediction system has learnt the life of wear law for the machine tools, as the RUL degradation pattern of the projected results is almost identical to the actual findings. The prediction accuracy is likewise strong, indicating that the prediction system has learnt the robot's and AGV's respective life degradation patterns.

9.5.2 The Result of AR-Assisted Upkeep

The outcomes of the machine tools, AGVs, and robot AR-assisted maintenance are shown in Figures 9.6–9.8, correspondingly. As seen in Figure 9.6, augmented reality helps with machine tool maintenance by superimposing a 3D representation of the tool over the damaged sections. The whereabouts and state of the broken components may then be ascertained by the maintenance staff using this data. Figure 9.7 displays the

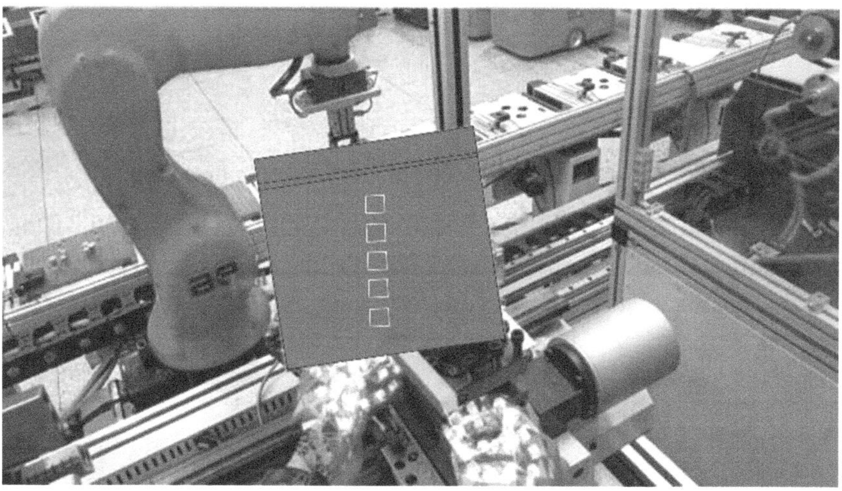

FIGURE 9.6 AR-based machine tool maintenance.

AGV's AR-assisted maintenance system, which uses augmented reality to incorporate visual maintenance recommendations into the real environment. AR assisted the maintenance crew to work on the AGV without removing it from its vehicle. Eliminating the need to read paper maintenance instructions, users may simply check off each step as they're done by clicking the "Finish" button. Figure 9.8 details the AR-assisted robot maintenance process, while the paper instructions detail the same process.

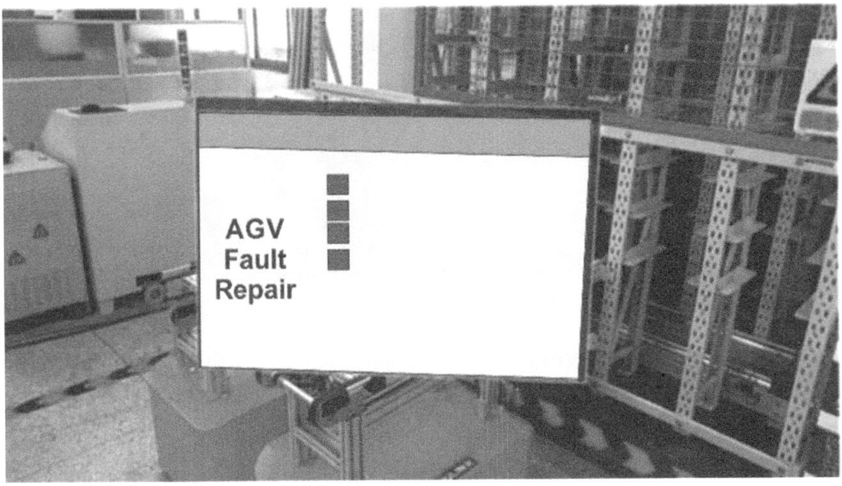

FIGURE 9.7 AR-based AGV maintenance.

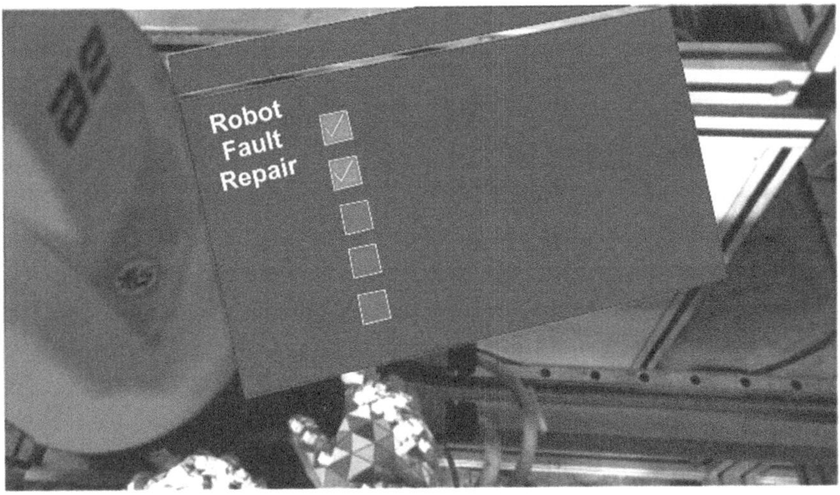

FIGURE 9.8 AR-based robot maintenance.

9.5.3 Remote Maintenance Using AR

Figure 9.9 illustrates that the remote expert's system is mostly used when the present work is more complex for the maintenance staff to handle technically and cannot be completed effectively. Employing the WebRTC protocol, the AR method establishes a video connection with a distant specialist in the local net. The issue is examined one step at a time under the direction of the remote specialist. To help the maintenance staff continue the repair process, the remote expert will notify them of the issue by annotation once they have identified it.

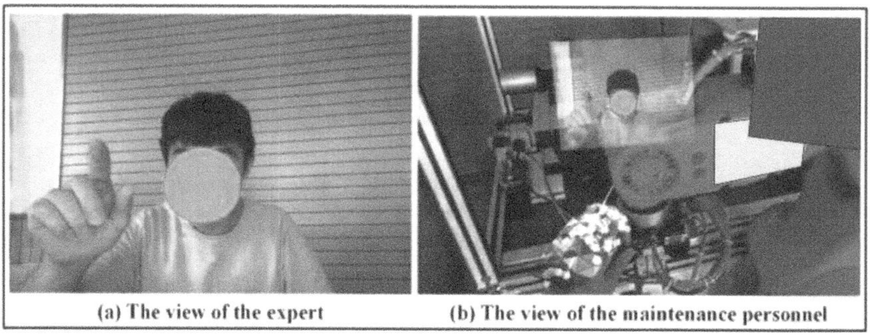

FIGURE 9.9 AR-based remote guidance. (a) The view of the expert and (b) the view of the maintenance personnel.

9.6 DISCUSSION

9.6.1 Comparison of RUL Prediction Accuracy

The accuracy of the predictions is to be determined by doing 100 experiments on each of the 20 randomly selected test samples. Compared to the other comparison algorithms, the suggested approach outperforms them in terms of RUL prediction accuracy. The results indicate that deep learning algorithms can outperform ELM when it comes to data association mining and fitting, as compared to conventional machine learning. One promising approach that has been discussed in the literature is a deep reinforcement learning-based system for scheduling the maintenance staff. However, the primary goal of accuracy work is to enhance the RUL algorithm's model structure so that the future maintenance plan may be based on a more realistic set of assumptions. Additionally, the aforementioned RUL method predicts outcomes for types of equipment that are different from than those tested in this study. Figure 9.10 shows that the proposed RUL prediction model has somewhat greater accuracy than the previously discussed technique in the study.

9.6.2 Advantages of Augmented Reality–Focused PHM

Figure 9.11 shows the benefits of AR-assisted PHM. AR-assisted management (the light line) takes less time than standard maintenance (the dark line). In case 1, the variation in the time needed for upkeep is significant because the job isn't difficult enough. In the third case, the variance in maintenance time is very large due to the complexity of the job at hand. Additionally, AR significantly improves the efficiency of maintenance by providing clear instructions, especially for difficult maintenance chores.

Algorithm	Average Accuracy
CNN	92.57%
CNN-GRU	95.62%
GRU	94.40%
ELM	90.38%
DNN	94.69%
ELSTMNN	95.13%
CNN-LSTM	95.28%
CNN-XGBoost	96.03%
CNN-BiLSTM	95.84%
Proposed System	98.17%

FIGURE 9.10 Precision of various systems.

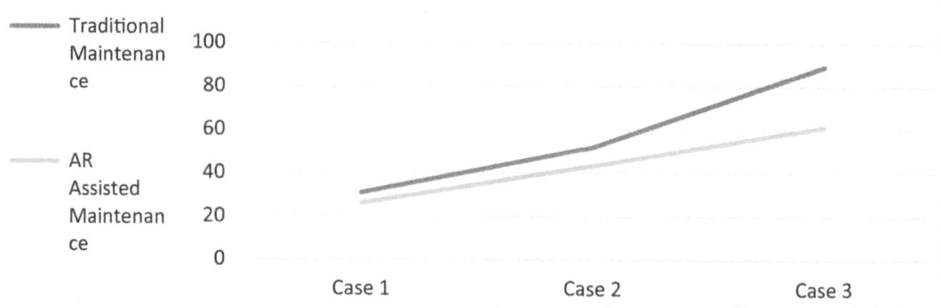

FIGURE 9.11 Benefits of AR-assisted PHM.

9.7 CONCLUSION

With the use of augmented reality and the Internet of Things, this research aims to develop a health management structure based on deep learning. The high-precision RUL prediction results are achieved, which are the foundation of reliable maintenance, by implementing a PSO convolution neural network. PSO achieves efficient feature extraction from large production information sets, and it finds the ideal value by initializing a set of particles and continuously revising their speed and location. To suit the RUL result, GRU attention is built on top of AR-assisted PHM to mine the relationships between these aspects. Users will pay more attention to important information because of the attention process. AR-assisted maintenance is used to help technicians see what they need to do depending on the predicted RUL result. The AR remote specialist can also provide advice in the form of annotations to help the maintenance staff keep working on the project. The experiment shows that this method is better than other ways of comparing things in terms of both accuracy and speed.

Eventually, the IOT-enabled factory will use a larger fleet of equipment. This chapter's suggested method necessitates the incorporation of the cloud-edge orchestration mechanism. It is possible to implement the RUL model for prediction on every industry computer of the edge machine tools and the method for scheduling maintenance staff in the cloud. AR allows for more accurate job assignments, which in turn improves maintenance efficiency and the assignment of relevant workers to those tasks.

BIBLIOGRAPHY

1. Patel, Mohit, et al. "Enhancing disaster response training through immersive AR/VR simulations." *2023 6th International Conference on Advances in Science and Technology (ICAST)*. IEEE, 2023.
2. Velev, Dimiter, and Plamena Zlateva. "Augmented and virtual reality application in disaster preparedness training for society resilience." *International Multidisciplinary Scientific GeoConference: SGEM* 18.4.3 (2018): 195–201.
3. Bhardhwaj, Tanav, and Tarun Kumar. "Innovative approach to urban disaster preparedness." *International Conference on Business and Technology*. Cham: Springer Nature Switzerland, 2024.
4. Khanal, Shishir, et al. "Virtual and augmented reality in the disaster management technology: a literature review of the past 11 years." *Frontiers in Virtual Reality* 3 (2022): 843195.
5. Surtiari, Gusti Ayu Ketut, et al. "Making virtual reality (VR)/augmented reality (AR) possible to strengthen disaster risk reduction among communities at risk of Tsunami." *International Journal of Disaster Management* 6.3 (2024): 291–312.
6. Sermet, Yusuf, and Ibrahim Demir. "Virtual and augmented reality applications for environmental science education and training." In Linda Daniela (ed) *New Perspectives on Virtual and Augmented Reality*. Routledge, 2020. 261–275.
7. BramahHazela, J. H., T. Rajasanthosh Kumar, S. Kavitha, D. Deepa, S. Lalar, and P. Karunakaran. "Machine learning: supervised algorithms to determine the defect in high-precision foundry operation." *Journal of Nanomaterials* 2022.1 (2022): 1732441.
8. Faiz, Tauqeer, et al. "A scoping review on hazard recognition and prevention using augmented and virtual reality." *Computers* 13.12 (2024): 307.
9. Kumar, A. "Smart agriculture using IoT." *International Journal of Innovative Research in Computer Science & Technology* 9.6 (2021): 188–191.
10. Rathore, P. S., S. Ahuja, S. R. Burri, A. Khunteta, A. Baliyan, & Kumar, A. (2024a). *Deep learning techniques for automation and industrial applications*. John Wiley & Sons, Inc.; Scrivener Publishing LLC.
11. Kao, Chia-Lung, et al. "The development of new remote technologies in disaster medicine education: a scoping review." *Frontiers in Public Health* 11 (2023): 1029558.
12. Sai Sanjana, K. B., K. Sai Mounika, T. Raja Santhosh Kumar, and D. V. Srikanth. "Thermal analysis of advanced IC engine cylinder." *International Journal of Automobile Engineering Research and Development (IJAuERD)* 6 (2016): 2277–4785.
13. Abbas, Jonathan R., et al. "Virtual reality in simulation-based emergency skills training: a systematic review with a narrative synthesis." *Resuscitation Plus* 16 (2023): 100484.

14. Anwar, Muhammad Shahid, et al. "Immersive learning and AR/VR-based education: cybersecurity measures and risk management." In Ahmed A. Abd El-Latif, Yassine Maleh, Mohammed A. El-Affendi, Sadique Ahmad (eds) *Cybersecurity Management in Education Technologies*. CRC Press, 2023. 1–22.
15. Scippo, Stefano, et al. "Innovative methodologies based on extended reality and immersive digital environments in natural risk education: a scoping review." *Education Sciences* 14 (2024): 1–33.
16. Obonyo, E. A., and L. A. Ouma. "Enhancing the resilience of low-income housing using emerging digital technologies." *IOP Conference Series: Earth and Environmental Science* 1101. 9 (2022).
17. Rathore, P. S., S. Ahuja, S. R. Burri, A. Khunteta, A. Baliyan, & A. Kumar, (2024). *Deep learning techniques for automation and industrial applications*. John Wiley & Sons, Inc.; Scrivener Publishing LLC.
18. Burov, O. Yu, et al. "ICT for disaster-resilient education and training." *Proceedings of the VII International Workshop on Professional Retraining and Life-Long Learning using ICT: Person-oriented Approach (3L-Person 2022)*. Virtual Event, Kryvyi Rih, Ukraine, October 25, 2022. No. 3482. CEUR Workshop Proceedings, 2023.
19. Fisher, Joshua A., ed. *Augmented and Mixed Reality for Communities*. CRC Press, Taylor & Francis Group, 2021.
20. Gräf, Miriam, Maren Mehler, and Sara Jourdan. "Crisis management in the metaverse: designing virtual worlds for real-world resilience." (2024). *ICIS 2024 Proceedings*. 3. https://aisel.aisnet.org/icis2024/iot_smartcity/iot_smartcity/3
21. Kourtesis, Panagiotis. "A comprehensive review of multimodal XR applications, risks, and ethical challenges in the metaverse." *Multimodal Technologies and Interaction* 8.11 (2024): 98.
22. Stanney, Kay M., et al. "Performance gains from adaptive eXtended Reality training fueled by artificial intelligence." *The Journal of Defense Modeling and Simulation* 19.2 (2022): 195–218.
23. Yaqoob, Ibrar, et al. "Metaverse applications in smart cities: enabling technologies, opportunities, challenges, and future directions." *Internet of Things* 23 (2023): 100884.
24. Higham, H., and B. Baxendale. "To err is human: use of simulation to enhance training and patient safety in anaesthesia." *BJA: British Journal of Anaesthesia* 119.suppl_1 (2017): i106–i114.
25. Yan, Wanglin, et al. "Developing the eXtended tangible user interface as an experimental platform for geo CPS." *Emerging Technologies for Disaster Resilience: Practical Cases and Theories*. Springer, 2021. 11–32.

CHAPTER 10

The Adoption of AR and VR Emergency Room Procedures

Swetha N, K. Madhavi, Rajiv U Kalebar, Anitha Nallasivam, and C Selvaraj

10.1 INTRODUCTION

Medical imaging has grown into a field that can create multidimensional, highly detailed 4D imagery. An important part of diagnosing and treating patients is being able to understand their complicated structure and disease. These days, preoperative image data is often used in oral and cranio-maxilla facial surgery (OCS), after which a 3D virtual surgery plan (VSP) is run through the data. Oral and maxillary surgeons, neurosurgeons, and trauma surgeons all employ 3D VSP to plot and forecast the outcomes of complex procedures. In modern oncology resection surgery, preoperative imaging is used to create a VSP. MRI data [3] can be utilized to help distinguish soft tissues, such as tumours, from bone structures. Cone-beam computed tomography (CBCT) data [2] is often used to plan the tumour-removal areas andI any necessary reconstruction [4]. Surgical guides and patient-specific plates made with computer-aided design and manufacturing (CAD/CAM) are often used to translate the VSP into a practical tool that can be used in the operating room. However, if the guides are not placed correctly, the surgery will not go as planned [5]. Surgical guides can't be used for soft parts or deep, narrow surgical methods. The employment of real-time tracking technologies is essential for the smooth

DOI: 10.1201/9781003564904-10

operation of the 3D VSP in the operating room. Both the patient's well-being and the surgical outcome are improved by imagery-guided surgery (IGS) technologies, which also help surgeons navigate the surgical environment. IGS has been shown to make it significantly easier for doctors to locate internal structures, reduce the duration of operations, and ease the surgeon's workload. During the procedure, image data can be linked to the patient as well as the tools for surgical guidance. A 3D virtual layout is made using image data (CT, MRI) to start the robotic surgery guidance process. The plan shows things like the edges of the incision, where the screws will go, and the outline of important internal structures. After that, the guidance device tells the patients about the surgery plan. Surgical guidance is based on the registration, which is done by connecting specified points on the image data to where things are. Surgical navigation provides real-time information to the surgeons on the optimal positioning of the surgical equipment relative to the patient's anatomy; they can see in real time how the instruments and image data are related in space. On the patient, virtual points or goals in the surgery plan can be found even if the surgeon is not there in person. With the use of augmented reality (AR) and the Internet of Things (IoT), this research aims to develop a health management system based on deep learning. We can achieve high-precision remaining useful life (RUL) prediction results, which are the foundation of reliable maintenance, by implementing PSO-CNNs (particle swarm optimization-convolutional neural networks). PSO achieves efficient feature extraction from large production data sets, and it finds the optimal value by initializing a set of particles and continuously revising their speed and position. Most of the images used in surgical navigation systems right now are shown on standard 2D panels. Surgeons usually have to look at the patient's information on the 2D monitors or screens that are fixed to the wall from a distance, and sometimes the screens are angled in a position that isn't the same as the surgery field. For this to work, the surgeons have to mentally analyze the imagery that has been seen and cast it onto the surgery field. This can be difficult, and doctors have to shift their eye, focus, and attention. It takes longer than necessary and makes mistakes more likely. Also, this kind of setting doesn't let the surgeon carefully look at the data while the surgery is going on, so a second person has to give the data indirectly. This kind of unclear interaction can negatively affect surgical outcomes, complicate the cleaning process, waste time, and increase the risk of sepsis. Mobile displays have been utilized to address some of these problems. These screens are attached to surgical instruments, helping to reduce surgery time and make medical navigation easier to learn. However, recent progress in technology has made augmented reality, or AR, by way of a head-mounted display (HMD) a method that can be used to fix these problems. AR's main benefit within operating rooms is that it lets doctors directly visualize spatial information in the real world by superimposing virtual images onto or near the patient's body. Additionally, gesture-based engagement methods can enable surgeons to work with patients and connect directly with imagery data. Another possibility for this kind of method is to give the surgeon more control, save time, and maintain a sterile environment.

AR is being looked at by surgeons in many fields, such as orthopaedics, spine surgery, neurology, laparoscopy, and biopsies. This chapter explains how AR systems can be applied in OCS for procedures such as post-trauma cosmetic surgery, orthodontic treatments, creal-time joint motion evaluation, sentinel node biopsy, and tumour removal. One system involved the development of a see-through display that does not require fixed localization systems, instead relying on coloured markers for visual tracking. This display is used in procedures involving orthognathic (jaw-related) treatment. Virtual surgical planning is overlaid onto the patient using a handheld display and is tracked through a surgical navigation system. The Microsoft HoloLens is proposed as a tool to help remove tumours during skull-base surgery, although it requires manual point-based registration. A brand-new guidance system that combines an AR interface with the Microsoft HoloLens is also introduced.

This study focuses on a device that enables the surgeon to view data from a camera positiond near the patient during surgery. This technique supports oncology-related procedures for OCS patients to conduct sterile pre- and postoperative discussions using 3D patient-specific planning and navigation data. The method aimed to facilitate the surgeon's visualization of the 3D VSP for the benefit of the patients, allowing for improved eye-hand coordination, quicker and more precise surgery, and greater visual feedback overall. During the operation, the surgeon's perspective was enhanced with the surgical plan and postoperative guidance data using the HoloLens device. Comparing the technique to traditional surgical methods proved its efficacy.

10.2 METHODS AND MATERIALS

10.2.1 Design of Systems

This section discusses the development of augmented reality systems that go beyond standard display technologies. The first step involved integrating a surgical navigation device, Brainlab, with the Microsoft HoloLens. The patient and navigation data could then be visualized in real time. The guidance system's data is displayed in 3D, and the operators can move it around as they see fit. In addition, the surgeon may interact with the 3D virtual surgical plan material by speaking voice commands or using predefined hand gestures.

10.2.2 Needs for the System

For a system to be useful in the hospital setting, it must work with the current process and not be worse than current methods. So, we made a list of all the design needs based on how surgery is currently done. This approach was designed with the following goals in mind:

- G1: Does not need any change to current surgical workflows or treatment practices
- G2: Recognize voice commands and hand motions and adjust the image to match
- G3: Allow for modification of the entire AR environment as well as specific items within it
- G4: Enable users to show or hide individual items
- G5: Support contextual and focused viewing
- G6: Improve head-hand alignment
- G7: Be easier to add on to
- G8: Be simple to use and take little time to learn

The technology is designed to assist the physician during surgical procedures. With this in mind, using the procedure shouldn't require a shift in current office practices (G1). Physicians can position the augmented reality content whenever it is most convenient for them. This eliminates the need for them to mentally keep track of multiple factors, such asthe individual undergoing surgery, the surgical strategy, the imaging data, and the procedural instructions (G3). Using hand gestures, surgeons can interact with the 3D image data without having to leave the sterile environment. Mostly, voice commands are used for some tasks that can't be easily incorporated into the visualization. Voice commands also keep the surgeons from leaving the work area (G2). Surgical strategies include a wide range of data, but if everything is viewed through the HoloLens, some important details may not be visible. To address this, the user can selectively hide or show individual components in our system (G4). At times, users may want to focus on and discuss a specific element. For example, doctors sometimes talk about the shape or structure of a tumour during the surgery. However, they generally prefer not to alter its actual position in the AR display. Researchers made this feasible by allowing users to duplicate components with a straightforward air tap (G5).

10.2.3 Surgery System Based on Images

Figure 10.1 shows an outline of the augmented reality image-guided surgery (ARIGS) device that was made. The system does three things: it obtains the surgery plan and navigation information from the navigation

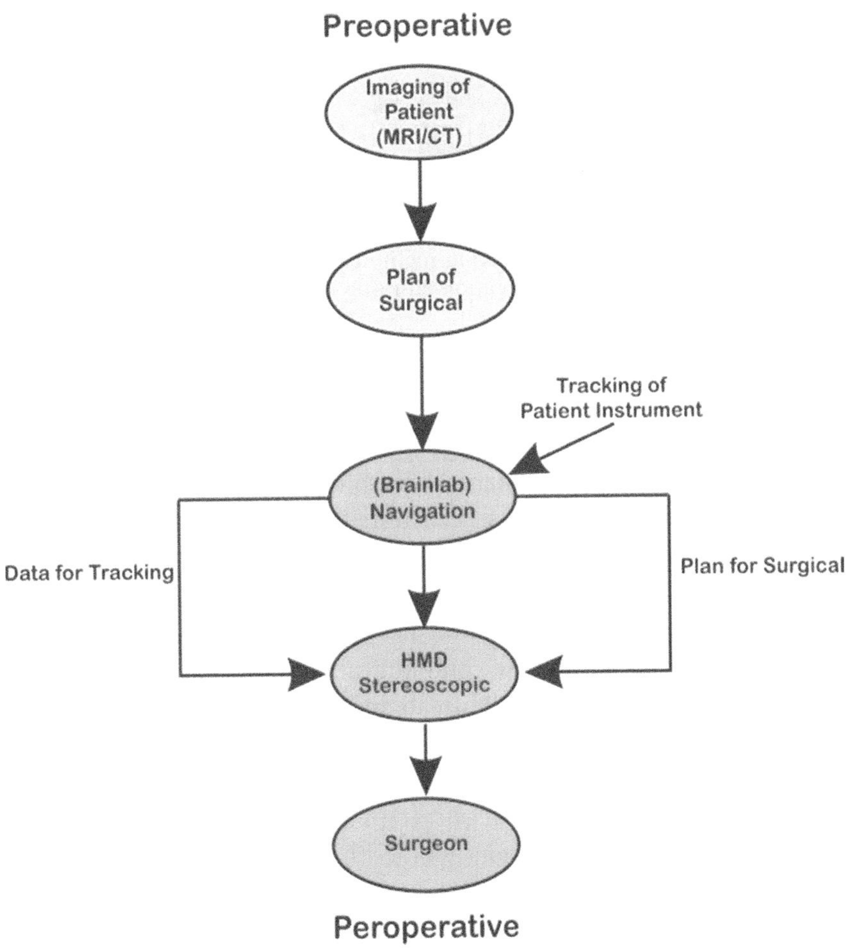

FIGURE 10.1 Overview of process.

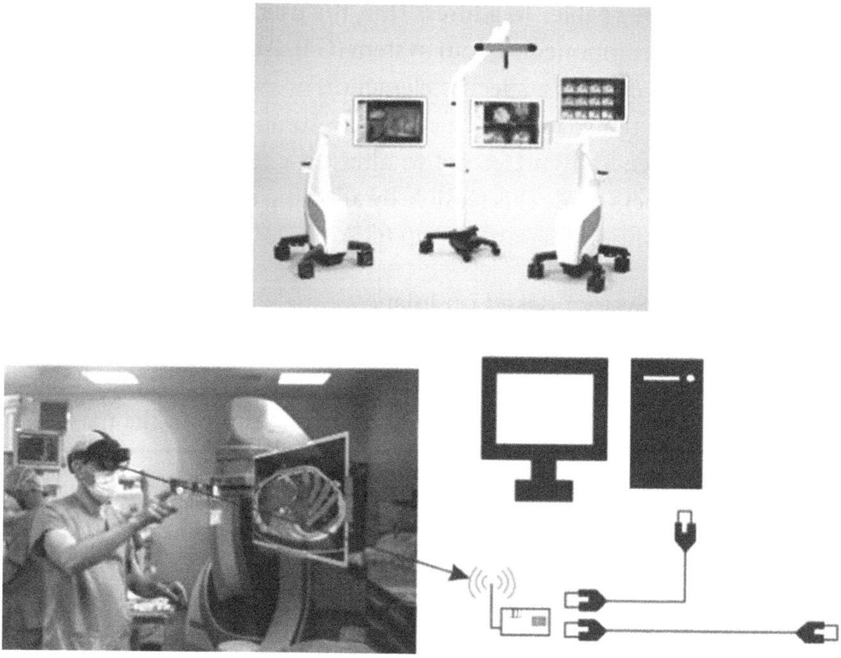

FIGURE 10.2 Hardware parts.
Top: Traditional Brainlab navigation method. Bottom Left: A surgeon wearing HoloLens. Bottom Right: Application-running PC. A dedicated router connects all gear.

gear, it processes the images, and it shows the surgeon the results. The hardware parts are shown in Figure 10.2. These include the widely available guidance system Brainlab, Microsoft's HoloLens, and a PC. The Brainlab guidance device has been tested and is utilized in clinics all over the world. When the surgery is complete, the PC gets the redefined VSP of the Brainlab along with tracking data from the medical tools. The Eyeopening system, an open-source net interface for guided image treatment that was created to ease communication between medical tools in the operating room, enables Brainlab and the PC to talk to each other. After the VSP is downloaded to the PC, binocular images are created and wirelessly transmitted to the HoloLens. The HoloLens has binocular, transparent screens that let the surgeon view both the surgical field and 3D virtual material simultaneously. Since the HoloLens is the same weight and size as a surgery headlight, it is comfortable to wear throughout the procdure. The wireless HoloLens gives the operator freedom of movement during surgery. It also lets you connect with data using voice commands and hand gestures while maintaining a sterile field. These hand movements and voice commands from the surgeon are sent back to the PC from the HoloLens. Based on what the user types in, the corresponding actions are processed, and the results are then displayed on the HoloLens.

The process begins with patient imaging and preoperative surgical (PS) plan correction. After that, the navigation system (Brainlab) loads and displays the surgical plan on the HMD.

10.2.4 Study of Users

The researcher conducted a comparison study to evaluate user performance and feedback with the method. Participants used a medical tool to complete some common navigation tasks on a custom-made phantom model. Brainlab's regular navigation interface was used as a standard, and the virtual reality interface was compared against it based on how fast, accurately, and qualitatively it replied to three research tasks.

10.2.5 Participants

People were asked to use both the regular navigation interface along with the virtual reality interface to complete several navigation tasks. After finishing all the tasks, the subjects were given an evaluation within the 5-point Likert scale to judge how useful the method was in terms of how easy it was to use, how accurate it was, how efficient it was, and how hard it was. The full evaluation is attached to this chapter as supplemental information. Under the number M19.225061, the medical integrity reviewing board of the University Therapeutic Center gave their permission for this project. All methods were carried out according to the rules and guidelines that were in place. Participants were properly informed, and their permission was gained after that.

10.2.6 Apparatus

As a test item for movement-related tasks, a 3D-printed phantom was used. To eliminate anatomical knowledge bias among experienced surgeon, the phantom was intentionally designed without any identifiable human body parts. This ensured that all participants had the same amount of information about the data and were not influenced by familiar physical details. A CBCT scan of the 3D dummy was generated and uploaded to the Brainlab preoperative guidance system. The researcher defined target locations and navigation paths that had to be found using the standard surgical guidance tool (Figure 10.3).

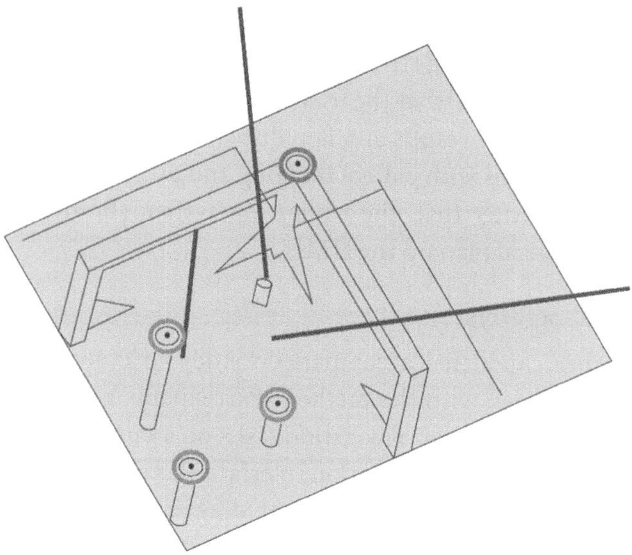

FIGURE 10.3 Duties and phantom. A 3D-printed phantom navigation activity with start point, three milestones, six floating landmarks and three trajectory jobs.

10.2.7 Tasks

Three actual markers and three motion-finding tasks were put to the test. The three physical landmark tasks consisted of a series of simple steps that had to be taken to locate the predefined physical landmarks on the phantom's structure. In this way, subjects received direct input when they finished the job. In trajectory finding tasks, participants were required to follow set paths, sometimes navigating around obstacles. According to the researcher, these paths were straight lines going in different directions that weren't parallel to any CBCT axis. This task was similar to planning a real surgery, like taking an established path to a tumour or putting in an implant. However, the six additional flying markers used in the trajectory task were treated as extra tests, and when they were reached, participants no longer received direct feedback.

As part of the tracking task, participants had to guide the instrument from one moving point to another, always staying on the planned path. Participants in both groups were given 10 minutes to practice using the device before the real test. The people who took the tests were instructed to perform the tasks quickly and accurately. At the beginning of each trial, participants were asked to set the instrument back to its initial position and were then allowed to visually locate the target. The trial could begin with the voice command "start" as long as the participant had clearly identified the goal location. The command "end" was used to conclude the task when the participants thought they had hit the goal. The actual position of the tool (the tip) was continuously recorded. It shows both the Brainlab interface and the AR interface in the image.

10.2.8 Measurements

The position of the tool's tip was continuously tracked throughout the tasks. To determine the accuracy of reaching a landmark, the Euclidean distance between the final position of the instrument's tip and the target landmark was calculated. The root-mean-square (RMS) of the straight-line distance between the actual path and the intended route was used to quantify the degree to which a participant deviated from the intended path. Users' performance in all three scenarios was compared using a Student's t-test. Each participant was recorded in each scenario using four fixed landmarks, ten moving landmarks, and seven motion measurements.

10.3 RESULTS

Twelve men from the nearby university hospital took part in the study. They completed all the preplanned navigation tasks on both systems, utilizing Brainlab either with or without the HoloLens and in random order. Seven of the 13 participants said they have used the tracking system before. Prior experience meant using it at least 11 times. Two of these six expert individuals said they used it every day. The other seven people who took part in the experiment said they had never used the tracking system before. Participants' ages ranged from 31 to 58 (with a median = 45) years old. New users' ages ranged from 23 to 32 (with a median = 27) years old. Six of the people who took part were doctors, and the others were medical students.

10.3.1 Time

In the HoloLens condition, all tasks were finished 1.72 times faster compared to the Brainlab condition ($P = 0.035$). However, foue of the subjects did better when they used the Brainlab. People using HoloLens were 1.88 times quicker than people using Brainlab ($P < 0.02$), and people using HoloLens were 1.75 times faster ($P = 0.026$) when doing real-world landmark tasks. It took experienced people ($M = 238.4$ s, SD = 93.7 s) about the same amount of time to finish as it did those who were new ($M = 216.9$ s, SD = 229.9 s, $P = 0.762$).

10.3.2 Accuracy

The precision was much better with HoloLens ($P < 0.002$), but not with the real landmarks ($P = 0.088$). When the HoloLens was used, deviations from the planned paths were smaller ($P < 0.002$). When it came to reaching the flying points ($P = 0.153$) or following the paths ($P = 0.632$), neither the expert nor the novice users showed any significant differences. With a mean of 1.47 mm and a standard deviation of 0.48 mm compared to 2.55 mm and a standard deviation of 3.07 mm for the experienced users, the new users got to the designated positions with less errors ($P = 0.043$). Loss of tracking was the same in both cases ($P = 0.22$), so there was no real difference. Figure 10.4 shows how well each job was done and how long it took.

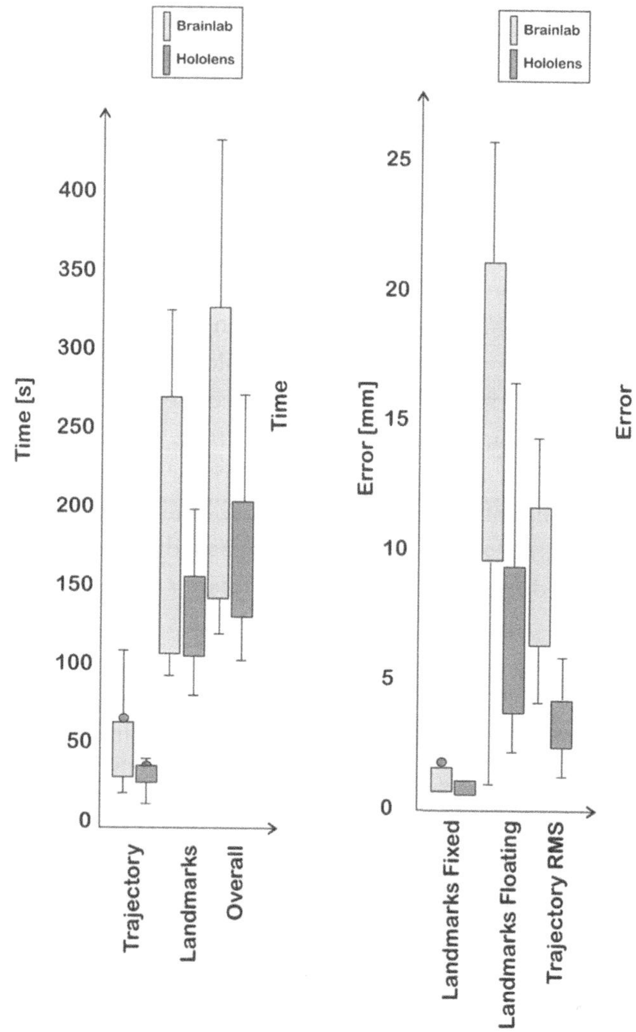

FIGURE 10.4 Mean, standard deviation, and 96% range of trust of three systems' navigation tasks.

Circles show mean values. HoloLens accuracy was substantially higher ($P < 0.002$), yet not for physical landmarks ($P = 0.088$). HoloLens reduced deviation from projected trajectory ($P < 0.002$).

The total length of the pathway was not significantly different between the two platforms ($P = 0.21$), but the HoloLens-based route was shorter when following the paths ($P = 0.036$). The scatter plots of how accurate the real and moving locations are can be seen in Figures 10.5 and 10.6.

Scatter plots of accuracy and route length following pathways are shown in Figures 10.7 and 10.8, respectively. As part of the post-lesson assessment, students were asked to choose which method they preferred. Although the participants had little knowledge of virtual reality/augmented reality (2.26/6 rating) and gesture-based interaction (3/6 rating), they said that using HoloLens simplified the tasks (3.26/6 score in Brainlab, 2.5/6 score in HoloLens). Goals G2 and G8, which deal with real-time experience, had an above-average rating for voice (3.7 out of 6), motions (2.9 out of 6), and the ease of understanding and following contact directions (3.8 out of 6).

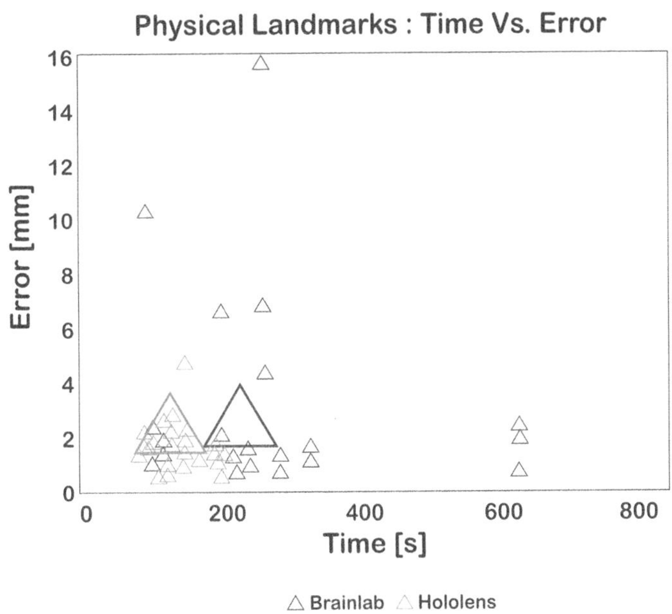

FIGURE 10.5 Time vs. landmark accuracy scatter plots.
Dark triangle: Brainlab, light triangle: HoloLens. Large triangles show mean values.

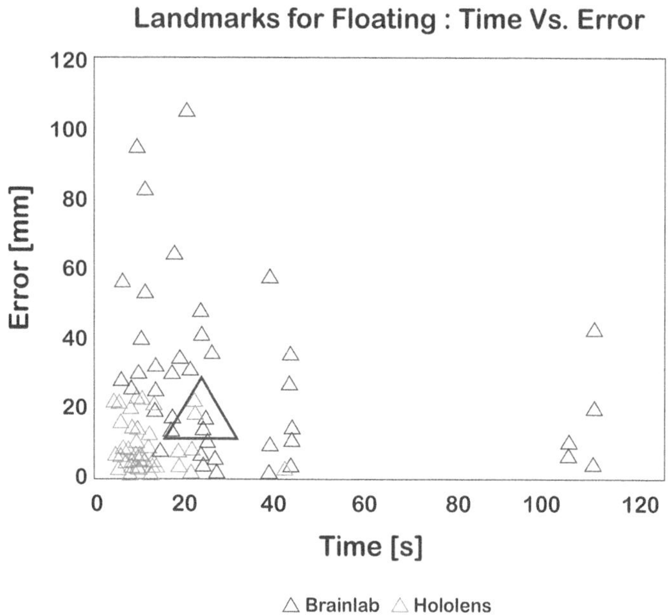

FIGURE 10.6 Time vs. floating landmark accuracy scatter plots.
Dark triangle: Brainlab, light triangle: HoloLens. Large triangles show mean values.

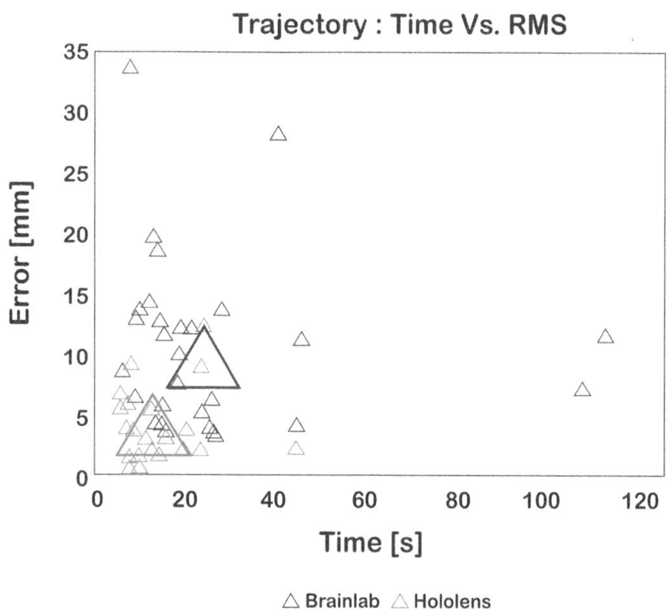

FIGURE 10.7 Trajectory-based time-accuracy scatter plots.
Dark triangle: Brainlab, light triangle: HoloLens. Large triangles show mean values.

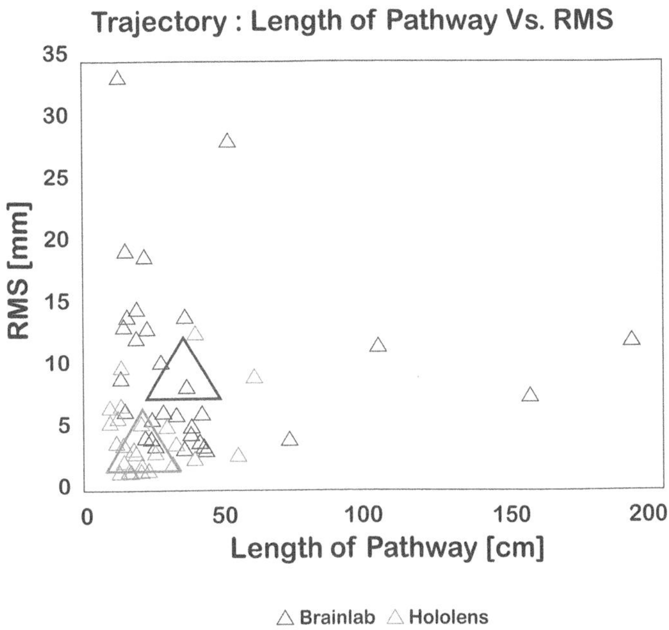

FIGURE 10.8 Scatterplots showing route length vs. trajectory accuracy. Dark triangle: Brainlab, light triangle: HoloLens. Large triangles show mean values.

10.3.3 Cases

The technique was first used during an oncology removal of an OCS patient. During a tonsillectomy followed by repair, guided surgery was used to find landmarks. Figure 10.9 offer a prime example of how a surgeon may use patient-specific data during an operation. Users could turn off motion inputs while working to keep the image from being changed without permission. With speech orders, they were able to save where the AR material was in space and how it was oriented. Due to the obstruction, the user has the option to reveal or conceal some elements. A duplicate of an object was shown alongside the original when an air trap was shown on single item.

The surgeon manually positions surgical visualization. Visualizing the desired goal enhances spatial orientation during tumour removal and reconstruction. For preoperative landmark recognition, navigation was utilized.

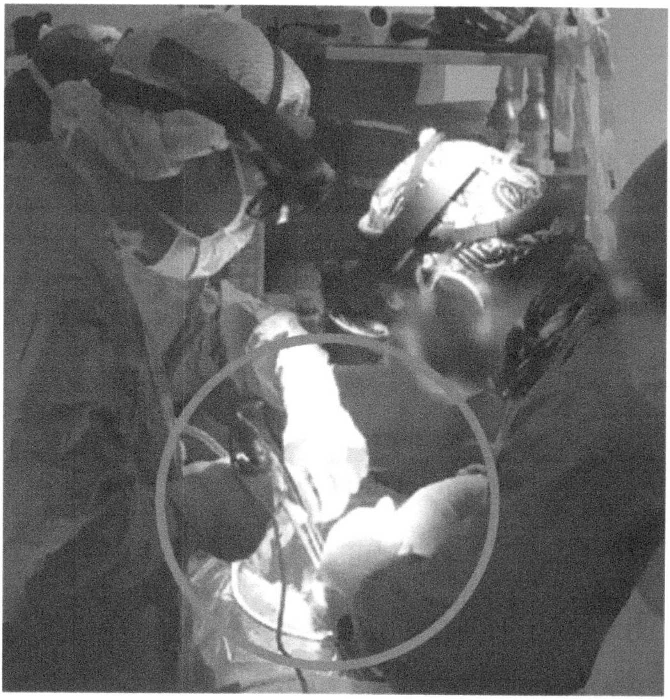

FIGURE 10.9 Utilized HoloLens to evaluate patient-specific surgical plans during CMF excision and repair.

10.4 DISCUSSION AND CONCLUSION

The researcher's technique for visualizing augmented reality makes navigation tasks more accurate and faster, especially the moving marker and trajectory tasks. Free-floating markers are a better way to show how to move through soft tissues in a clinical setting. Augmented reality representation makes eye-hand coordination better because it reduces deviation from trajectory tasks. This could mean less damage to tissues. It has been suggested that the Microsoft HoloLens might be utilized to help remove tumours during surgery on the base of the brain. However, to overlay virtual content, they used a human point-based registration method without validating its accuracy against the gold standard. In contrast, Brainlab is considered the industry leader. It offers a proven and accurate method that integrates directly with the HoloLens visualization system. Our system requires no additional registration procedures between the virtual and physical environments; it relies solely on input from the tracking equipment. We think this is an effective and secure method that minimizes the introduction of additional errors. In other tests, the HoloLens has been shown to work well in minimally invasive surgery, where it is used as a replacement for regular monitors. While the HoloLens has been useful, it's only used for 2D displays without tracking data. Another study reported on a brand-new guidance system that includes an augmented reality interface. The systems performance was judged by how accurately it placed an item in its intended location. However, the use of AR led to increased navigation errors because they relied on how well the virtual material lined up with the real world. The main difference between our study and theirs is that we did not attempt to align a 3D-printed item with the help of virtual images. Instead, we assessed the accuracy of the Brainlab system's verified pointer. Researchers believe this accounts for the difference in our results; researchers demonstrated that the use of the HoloLens made things more accurate.

Researchers receive the guidance data through the Brainlab system and transmit it into the HoloLens without relying on virtual material being superimposed on real-world objects. Piecrust et al. created an AR guidance system that could be used to cut bone in a fake jaw utilizing a digitally projected saw. Their "simple AR" approach is similar to the method used in this study in that it is based on tracking data instead of precise positioning and visual direction of the AR content. Their accuracy involves the tracking system's registration error, but with three control points, they achieved an average accuracy of 1.78 mm (§0.83 mm) and 1.89 mm (¥1.06 mm). We found the same level of accuracy when we used fixed landmarks: 1.77 mm (¥0.89 mm) for the experienced group along with 1.37 mm (¥0.45 mm) for the untrained group. However, using a biologically shaped phantom could make users less accurate, and the navigated saw could be more accurate if it were physically guided during the mastectomy procedure.

For the actual marker tasks, the HoloLens was faster, but not by a large amount. One reason for this could be that the test dummy was square and was scanned so that its form lined up with the digitalis, diagonal, and coronal axes. This might make it easier for the Brainlab user to coordinate their eyes and hands. Another possibility is that the players received physical input from the instrument once they located the marker. However, this isn't always how things work in real life, especially when the tracking goal is in soft tissue. During this trial, the Brainlab guidance system was also directly given to the participants, which won't always be possible in a hospital setting. Inexperienced users were better at getting to set points, no matter what technique they used. During surgery, the rate of loss tracking is important. When the navigation system loses track of the patient or the tool, doctors usually turn their attention from the patient to the navigation system. Still, there was no significant difference between the two conditions when it came to loss of tracking, though some participants did experience an 8.5% drop in the HoloLens condition. To support image-guided surgery, we developed a system that integrates virtual reality. Our system allows users to visualize and interact with a virtual surgery plan along with tracking data on phantom model, and we believe it will work just as well in the operating room. Our method makes it easier for the surgeon to coordinate his or her eyes and hands in the operating room (G6) and lets them move around in the AR world and interact with specific items (G3 and G4). Users can make a copy of an object that is centred and change it with a simple "air-tap" motion (G5). We conducte worked compared to the traditional approach to setting up the surgical system. The results demonstrated that our new method is more accurate and faster at tracking tasks. Additionally, user surveys provided positive feedback.

As an alternative to already-tested image guidance techniques (G1 and G7), the process shown here can be utilized for a many different image-guided treatments. The next step in this project is to connect the surgery plan to the patient's actual operating site. This will turn it into a fully augmented reality-driven guidance system. A method like this can reduce and improve visual input, which could make the surgeon's job easier and help them better coordinate their eyes and hands. In the end, this study showed how an AR display system that has been tested can improve image-guided surgery. To sum up, AR improves the 3D process by making things more accurate and cutting down on time.

BIBLIOGRAPHY

1. Dinh, Alana, et al. "Perceptions about augmented reality in remote medical care: Interview study of emergency telemedicine providers." *JMIR Formative Research* 7 (2023): e45211.
2. Yoo, Suyoung, et al. "Adoption of augmented reality in educational programs for nurses in intensive care units of tertiary academic hospitals: mixed methods study." *JMIR Serious Games* 12.1 (2024): e54188.
3. Rathore, P. S., S. Ahuja, S. R. Burri, A. Khunteta, A. Baliyan, & A. Kumar (2024). *Deep learning techniques for automation and industrial applications.* John Wiley & Sons, Inc.; Scrivener Publishing LLC.
4. Wu, Tzu-Chi, and Chien-Ta Bruce Ho. "A scoping review of metaverse in emergency medicine." *Australasian Emergency Care* 26.1 (2023): 75–83.
5. Wang, Mengying, et al. "Method and application of information sharing throughout the emergency rescue process based on 5G and AR wearable devices." *Scientific Reports* 13.1 (2023): 6353.

6. Bond, William F., et al. "The use of simulation in emergency medicine: a research agenda." *Academic Emergency Medicine* 14.4 (2007): 353–363.
7. Kumar, T. Rajasanthosh, et al. "Quantitatively examines the feasibility of different configurations of the aftermarket supply chain enabling additive manufacturing." *Solid State Technology* 63.5 (2020): 492–507.
8. McGrath, Jillian L., et al. "Using virtual reality simulation environments to assess competence for emergency medicine learners." *Academic Emergency Medicine* 25.2 (2018): 186–195.
9. Warner, Leah S. Honigman, et al. "The most crowded US hospital emergency departments did not adopt effective interventions to improve flow, 2007–10." *Health Affairs* 34.12 (2015): 2151–2159.
10. Gao, Evangeline, et al. "Adoption of emergency department–initiated buprenorphine for patients with opioid use disorder: secondary analysis of a cluster randomized trial." *JAMA Network Open* 6.11 (2023): e2342786.
11. Lynn, Stephan G., and Arthur L. Kellermann. "Critical decision making: managing the emergency department in an overcrowded hospital." *Annals of Emergency Medicine* 20.3 (1991): 287–292.
12. Mewada, S., et al. "Research article smart diagnostic expert system for defect in forging process by using machine learning process. *System (In Section 4)* 19 (2022): 21.
13. Hajjarsaraei, Hedieh, Babak Shirazi, and Javad Rezaeian. "Scenario-based analysis of fast track strategy optimization on emergency department using integrated safety simulation." *Safety Science* 107 (2018): 9–21.
14. Hakimzada, A. Forogh, et al. "The nature and occurrence of registration errors in the emergency department." *International Journal of Medical Informatics* 77.3 (2008): 169–175.
15. Ricciardi, Carlo, et al. "Implementation and validation of a new method to model voluntary departures from emergency departments." *Mathematical Biosciences and Engineering* 18.1 (2021): 253–273.

CHAPTER 11

Improving Medical Diagnosis with Augmented Reality Visualization

Thulasi Bikku, Govinda Rajulu G, Pramoda Patro, and Kiran Sree Pokkuluri

11.1 INTRODUCTION

Augmented reality is a technique that allows computer-generated material to be superimposed on top of the actual environment [1]. Some examples of this kind of material include images, videos, music, text, and even 3D (three dimensional) objects [2–4]. A person's awareness and comprehension of their environment may be greatly improved with the help of these enhancements. Many industries such as marketing, e-commerce, entertainment, and education are now making more use of this technology [5]. Educational settings have seen a steady rise in the use of augmented reality technologies.

Augmented reality has numerous uses. Museums and astronomy classes are two examples of places that often employ AR for discovery-based learning [6–8]. Additionally, interactive learning experiences and three-dimensional presentations may enhance book material. Another area where augmented reality might be useful is in skill training, such as when teaching people how to fix airplanes [9]. Motive, greater enjoyment,

DOI: 10.1201/9781003564904-11

and focus are just a few of the advantages that students may receive from studying in augmented reality settings [10].

The World Health Organization reports that cardiovascular diseases (CVDs) account for an estimated several million fatalities annually [11], making them the leading cause of mortality globally. Therefore, the anatomical features and functions of the heart should be thoroughly explored by the world's future doctors [12]. As this organ is not easy to show, a graphic depiction might help with comprehension.

This chapter details the process of creating an Android app named Cardio Sim that improves students' knowledge of the heart and its maladies by addressing certain learning goals. A variety of heart failure conditions may be easily and interactively distinguished using the 3D heart object [13–15]. In addition, Cardio Sim enables the student to evaluate the results of the specified learning objectives. In its simplest form, this software aids users by displaying, via augmented reality, the architecture of the heart's blood flow [16]. On top of that, it uses augmented reality to assess students' ability to recognize heart failure in various settings utilizing various forms and sounds of heartbeats [17]. Atrial stenosis, mitral incompetence, and a normal heart are the three cardiac scenarios shown by Cardio Sim [18]. Learners may also use the app's self-assessment features to see how well they're doing in relation to the learning objectives [19]. With this software, students may learn more about two different types of heart diseases [20–22]. Use of the System Usability Scale (SUS) and code testing were used to assess the Cardio Sim app's usability in this ADR [23].

11.2 RELATED WORKS

This section explores mobile apps with functionality comparable to Cardio Sim. Today, smartphones are widely available and play a significant role in people's lives [24]. Mobile apps have been developed to assist medical students in their study [25]. But a small number make use of augmented and virtual reality tools to improve education [26]. Some well-liked apps that people may find on the App Store and on Google Play are:

1. **Augmented Reality Anatomy 4D+ Program**:

   This app's standout features are its comprehensive translation into several languages and its augmented reality technology, which provides animated pictures of the major internal organs.

2. **My Organ Anatomy:**

   Using 3D images, this software shows the human body's internal structures. Plus, it has voice pronunciations for all medical terminology, lets users sketch on a blank screen and share screenshots, and more.

3. **My Heart Anatomy**:

   The software not only offers audio pronunciations of all phrases relevant to cardiac anatomy, but it also lets users choose any exterior portion of the heart to see its name and read associated information.

The Cardio Sim app was compared to the aforementioned apps, as summarized in Table 11.1. For instance, it's obvious that AR Anatomy 4D+ can't simulate organ disorders, and neither My Organ Anatomy nor My Heart Anatomy provides augmented reality features. While all three serve an instructional purpose, the clinical Skills and Simulation centre's semi-structured interviews led Cardio Sim to include the AR feature of self-assessment.

TABLE 11.1 Cardio Sim App Compared with Other Apps

Resources	**1.**	**2.**	**3.**	**Cardio Sim**
Usage of AR	Agree	Disagree	Disagree	Agree
Main Body Organs Coverage	Agree	Agree	Disagree	Disagree
My Organ Anatomy	Agree	Disagree	Agree	Disagree
Simulating and explaining	Disagree	Disagree		Agree
Giving information about organ	Disagree	Disagree	Agree	Agree
Organ parts audio pronunciation	Disagree	Agree	Agree	Disagree
Self-Evaluation	Disagree	Disagree	Disagree	Agree

11.3 MEDICAL SKILLS SIMULATION CENTRE AND CARDIO SIM APP OVERVIEW

The Cardio Sim app for Android devices incorporates augmented reality (AR) with medical education in an interactive way. To better educate students, it employs augmented reality in medical simulation. In spite of having less time in class, students may utilize it to keep up with real-world case training. More effective learning may be achieved with the use of AR and 3D objects that mimic various scenarios. With the use of case reports of heart failure, this app teaches users about the anatomy of the heart. Both mitral incompetence and mitral stenosis are cardiac failure scenarios covered by Cardio Sim. For each instance, it plays an instructional video that explains the symptoms and what causes them.

In order to practice on one of the manikins kept in the simulation and medical care skills centre, the Cardio Sim program will be used. Training possibilities in state-of-the-art technology skills are available at the clinical competence centres and simulation centre for those working in the healthcare, nursing, and allied health sectors. Actors playing the role of patients and computerized manikins that simulate sickness are two of the instructional tools used at the centre. In a safe environment, the centre offers opportunities to get practical experience. There are low-fidelity, medium-fidelity, and high-fidelity manikins at the centre.

The degree to which these manikins mimic reality determines which of the three groups they fall into. Several semi-structured interviews were carried out with the centre's personnel in order to determine the primary needs and app functionalities. They stressed the need to include material on heart failure as it is a foundational skill for students to acquire. Causes, symptoms, heart sounds, cardiac drawings, and blood flow are the learning outcomes requested by the cardiologists. Every one of these learning goals related to cardiac problems is addressed by the Cardio Sim program. The interviewers also recommended including a self-evaluation feature in the app.

11.4 METHODOLOGY

The process of organizing, creating, testing, and releasing a software project is known as software development methodology. Software development methodologies vary, but the most popular one is agile, which means it can both create and react to changes. As a strategy, it helps one cope with and ultimately thrive in a challenging and unpredictable setting.

Problematic formalization and producing and assessing the information technology object are the first two processes of ADR that we concentrated on while developing Cardio Sim. In order to manage the product via user involvement throughout development, the creators of the Cardio Sim app adopted the Scrum methodology, an agile framework.

There are two epics in the Cardio Sim app. The first epic's storylines include creating the application's pages and features, including the self-evaluation puzzles for each instance. The other epic delves into topics that pertain to the practical applications of augmented reality in cardiac problems and anatomy. Additionally, it has the features of case-specific self-evaluation exams.

11.4.1 Design of the Cardio Sim App

Use case, process, and sequence diagrams were among the many tools we used to examine the program throughout the project lifetime. As illustrated in Figure 11.1, the Cardio Sim app's two primary processes are

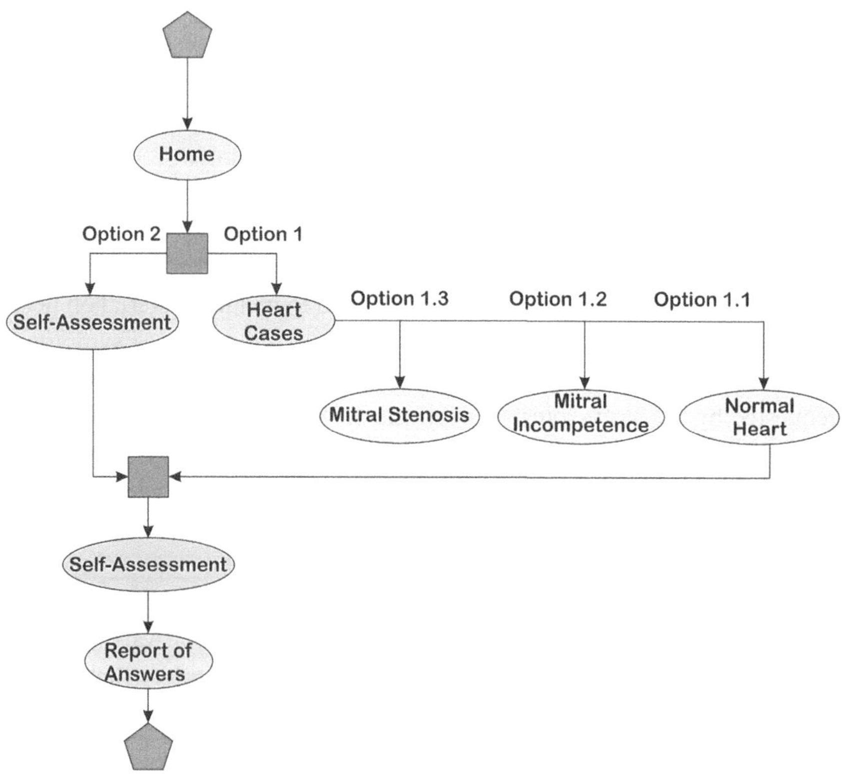

Figure 11.1 Cardio Sim app's two primary processes flow diagram.

shown using a system flow diagram. The app's components are described in detail in the following subsections:

11.4.1.1 Heart Cases

When the user selects the first option, heart cases are shown. There are a total of three sub-cases.

- The normal heart is shown when the operator chooses the heart cases menu. It will show the structure and function of a normal heart.
- The mitral incompetence case is shown when the operator picks it from the heart cases menu.
- Mitral stenosis instance is shown when the user selects cardiac cases, followed by the mitral stenosis instance.

11.4.1.2 Self-Assessment

The second option, self-assessment, initiates a quiz anytime the user selects it.

11.4.2 Implementation

The Cardio Sim app was developed using a variety of software technologies. Researchers began by using Vuforia Engine, a technology that facilitates the integration of powerful computer vision capabilities into augmented reality apps. This paves the way for picture recognition and real-world interaction inside the app. Second, we used Unity, a platform for creating augmented reality, virtual reality, and mixed reality applications. The third step was to develop the app's code in visual studio using the C# programming language. The fourth step was to utilize Android Studio, a tool that helps with app extraction from Unity and uploading it to Android-powered mobile devices.

The necessary hardware for this application consists of three parts:

1. A webcam, which helps with app testing and development;
2. A smart phone that focuses its camera at the manikin to illustrate its heart structure;
3. A manikin, which can be found and borrowed from the medical skills centre or virtual reality centre (see Figure 11.2).

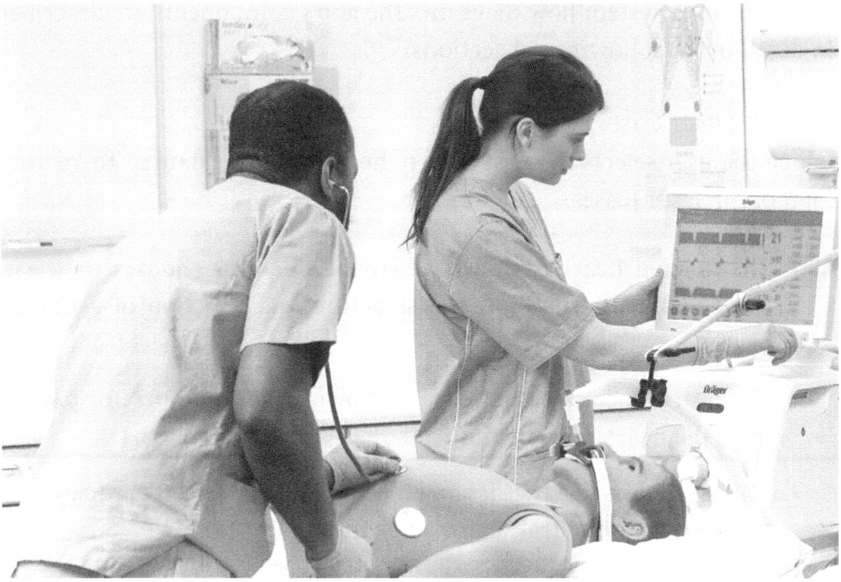

FIGURE 11.2 Cardio Sim Manikin in simulation centre.

11.5 ANALYSIS OF RESULTS AND EVALUATION

Three methodologies were used to test and assess the app: SUS, code testing, and usability testing. These methods were used to enhance the Cardio Sim app's usability and code quality.

11.5.1 Testing for Usability

While making Cardio Sim, the team utilized three of Nielsen's criteria for user crossing point plan.

- Every page of Cardio Sim follows the first rule of consistency: the buttons are always in the same places, and the colour palette is always the same. Regardless of the kind of self-assessment or cardiac situation, the operator will always follow a similar series of steps.
- The second guideline is to make it easy for regular users to utilize keyboard shortcuts. The regulation is enforced by making the help page accessible in more than one manner. Either the menu button or the "Cardio Sim" image at the top of every page may be used to access the homepage.
- Thirdly, we made sure to accommodate the user's internal point of control when we designed the app interface. Users are able to control

the sounds in Cardio Sim. Thus, the program may be silenced whenever the user chooses. The Cardio Sim app's usability was enhanced to better meet users' needs by including these principles throughout the design process.

11.5.2 Testing the Code

Two metrics, unit testing and integration testing, are used to appraise the code. Unit testing was conducted once each individual story was completed since this application was built using Scrum methodology. As an example, Cardio Sim has been tested to ensure that the following features are accessible: main menu, self-assessment, homepage navigation, answer choices self-assessment response report display, mitral incompetence, 3D heart, stenosis objects, and heartbeat on/off functionality.

Last but not least, we made sure that the user may start and pause all heart-related videos and the quiz. There were no negative outcomes, and the user was able to successfully finish every scenario. Consistent integration testing is key to guaranteeing a bug-free system. Making sure Cardio Sim is implemented properly requires running both measures of code testing.

The proper flow across screens is shown by the integration testing. Figure 11.3(a) depicts the home page; Figure 11.3(b) illustrates the menu that appears when the user clicks on the icon. In order to access the help feature, the user may either go to the menu or click on the help symbol.

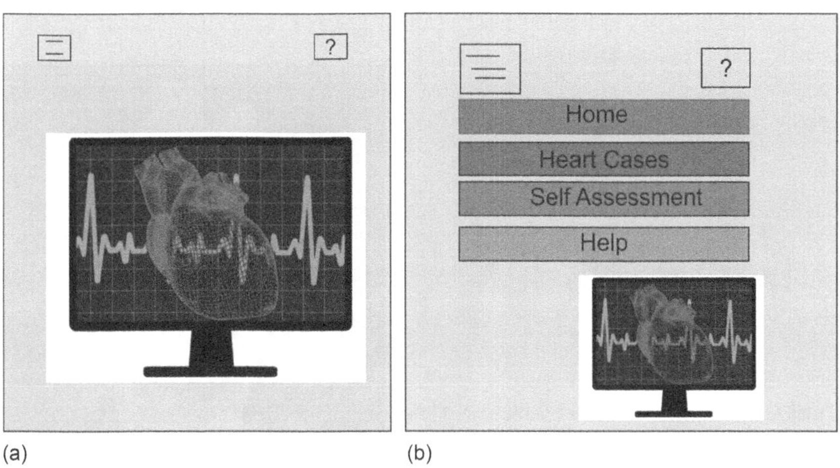

FIGURE 11.3 (a) Home page (b) menu that appears when the user clicks on the icon.

Although they vary in substance, the heart cases have a common design. The heart might be considered normal, mitral incompetent, or mitral stenosis. A 3D heart object customized for each case will be seen on the manikin when the user points the camera in that direction; simultaneously, the app will play the sound of the selected case's heartbeat.

As demonstrated in Figure 11.4(a) and (b) for the normal heart, Figure 11.5(a) and (b) for mitral incompetence, and Figure 11.6(a) and (b) for mitral stenosis, the user can access more detailed information about the selected case by clicking on the "show more" option on the heart cases page.

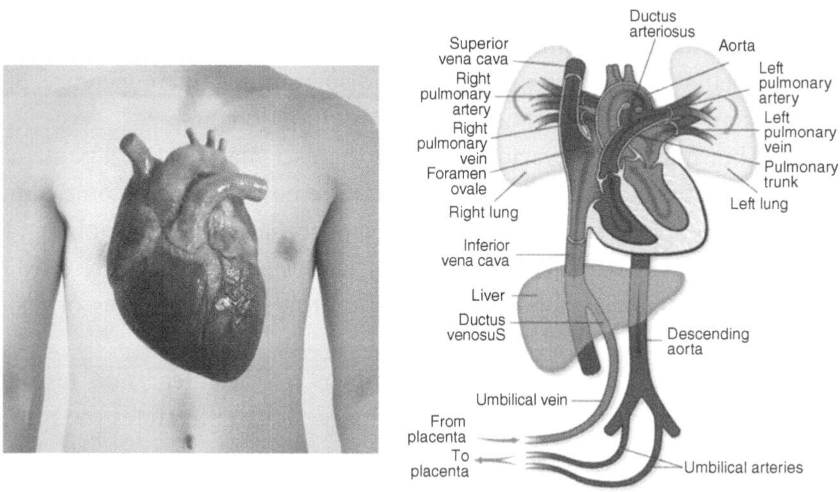

FIGURE 11.4 (a) and (b) Normal heart.

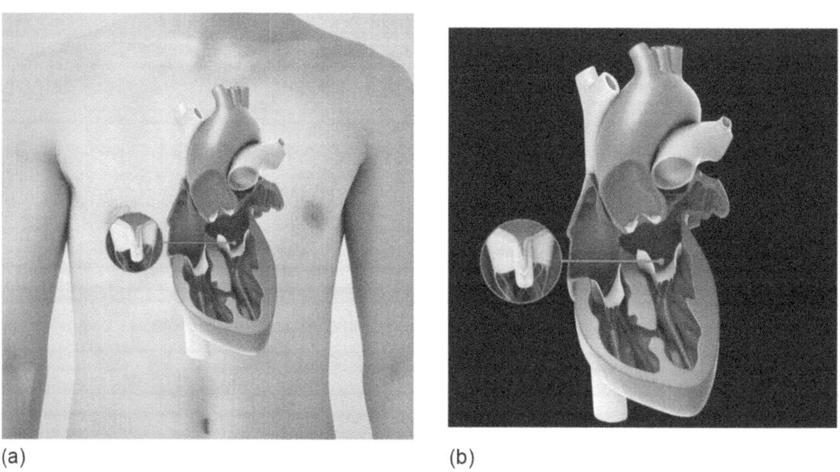

(a) (b)

FIGURE 11.5 (a) and (b) Mitral incompetence.

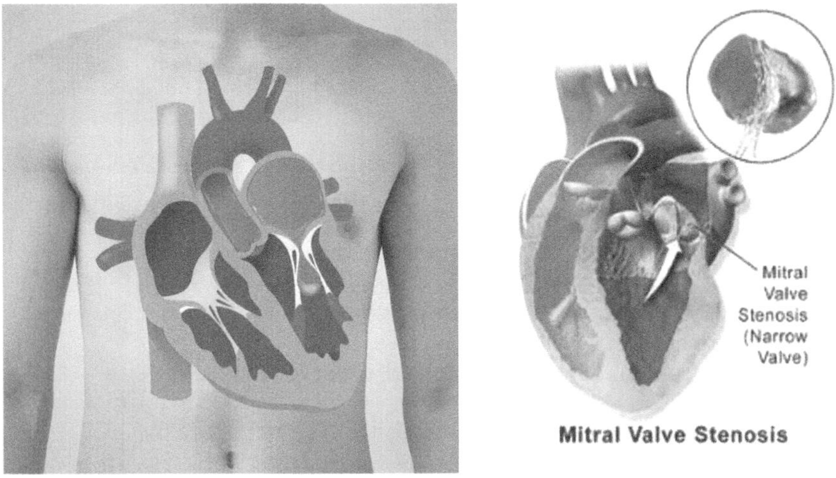

(a) (b)

FIGURE 11.6 (a) and (b) Mitral stenosis.

Additionally, each page has three alternatives at the bottom. The first choice is to activate or deactivate the heartbeat sound. The alternative is to begin viewing the informational film that provides further details on the selected instance, including the description of symptoms and causes. The third choice is to initiate a self-assessment quiz that encompasses the user's acquired knowledge during the session. Conducting tests in this manner enables us to examine and understand how the Cardio Sim app handles transactions between various components. All of the epics were successfully tested.

11.5.3 SUS

An instrument that measures the perceived usefulness of a system or technology is the System Usability Scale (SUS), and it serves as one of the most often used. Its creator, John Brooke, was engaged in digital equipment work. The survey asks respondents to score their degree of agreement with ten items. There are half positive and half negative wordings on the examinations. The agreements are evaluated using a five-point scale. The Cardio Sim app's usability was evaluated using SUS. Using a combination of convenience and snowball sampling, researchers were able to enlist ten centre-based medical students as participants. This data analysis yielded an acceptable SUS score of 77.76, placing it in the excellent category according to the SUS grading scale.

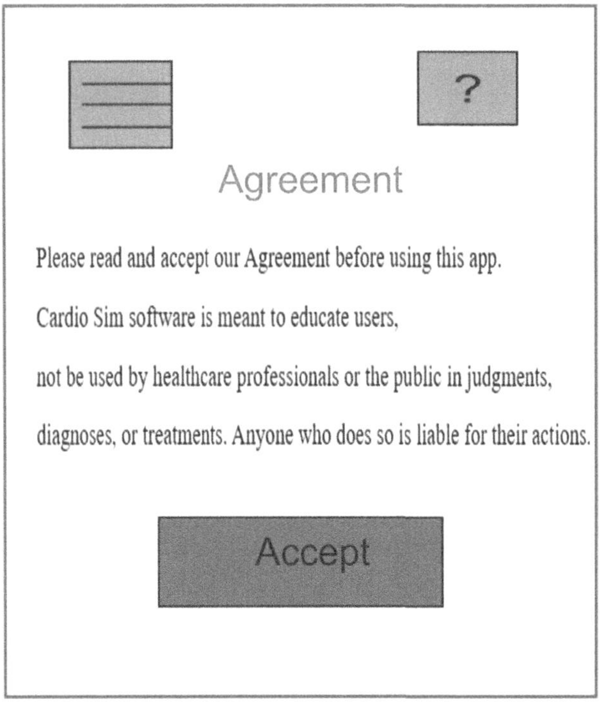

FIGURE 11.7 Release of responsibility agreement page.

11.5.4 Liability Release

A legal document known as a release of responsibility agreement is entered into between two parties when one party promises not to sue the other. This release of responsibility agreement is part of the Cardio Sim app and was created by us to prevent any potential abuse (see Figure 11.7).

11.6 DISCUSSION WITH LIMITATIONS

Research conducted by the Medical Skills as well as Virtual Reality Centre on the use of Cardio Sim in medical education shows that AR has great promise as a tool to improve learning. Students have a new tool at their disposal with augmented reality technologies: a dynamic and interactive approach to engage with complicated medical subjects. Users are able to better comprehend a variety of cardiac problems with the usage of Cardio Sim, which simulates cardiac architecture and heart failure instances.

Immersive learning using many heart failure scenarios and aural representations of distinct heartbeats improves retention and understanding. Students of medicine may greatly benefit from these additions as they provide more accurate and realistic depictions of real-world clinical scenarios. The positive comments from the usability test suggests that Cardio Sim has excellent usability and user acceptability, as it has been well-received by professionals. The emphasis here was on usability, although Cardio Sim does show promise as an AR-based medical teaching tool. Additional study is needed to fully understand the app's influence on medical knowledge retention and student learning outcomes; this review just scratches the surface.

11.6.1 Limitations

The study had a number of limitations, one of which is that the assessment was limited to the Cardio Sim app's usability. While the system usability scale did a good job of gauging how happy users were with the app's design and overall usability, it failed to evaluate the app's usefulness as a learning tool for medical students. A combination of qualitative and quantitative methodologies should be used in future assessments to evaluate learning outcomes, such as students' ability to apply the ideas in real-life clinical situations, and how the app affects their knowledge acquisition and retention.

Furthermore, the results cannot be applied to a broader population due to the tiny size of the usability testing group. The app's functioning and usefulness across various user types may be better understood if the user base is expanded to include a wider and more varied set of medical professionals and trainees.

A further limitation is that the ADR approach is not fully implemented. So far, the research has only covered the groundwork for the challenge and the construction of IT artifacts. In order to grasp the project's larger significance, the reflection as well as the formalization of learning stages must be finished. Therefore, the final thoughts and takeaways from the project, which might help with the app's improvement and future updates, are still in the works.

11.7 FUTURE WORK

An expansion of the assessment phase to more thoroughly examine the app's instructional success should be the focus of future development on Cardio Sim. This can include following up with students and healthcare workers over time to see how the app affects their ability to remember information, make diagnoses, and make decisions. In order to guarantee accurate and trustworthy results, the assessment should use tried-and-true methods for measuring learning outcomes. In the absence of such a tool, it may be worthwhile to create and validate an evaluation instrument tailored to AR medical simulations.

To further improve the app and its execution, it is necessary to carry out the remaining ADR steps, which include analysis and formalization of learning. During these steps, you may assess the study's strengths and weaknesses, pinpoint its improvement areas, and derive judgments on the app's larger implications for medical education. Iterative development relies on including input from learners and professionals who use the application in clinical settings.

Additionally, Cardio Sim might be expanded to include a broader spectrum of cardiovascular disorders and other medical issues, not limited to only heart failure situations. As a result of this growth, medical schools may have access to a more robust resource. A more immersive experience and more detailed engagement with the heart and its circumstances might be achieved by incorporating additional augmented reality technologies, such as haptic feedback or more complex 3D modelling.

11.8 CONCLUSION

In conclusion, the Cardio Sim application is an encouraging step forward in the field of medical education's use of augmented reality. The app's capacity to mimic cardiac architecture, heart failure scenarios, and related symptoms makes it a cutting-edge and useful educational resource that improves comprehension via dynamic and engaging activities. The app's promising performance in usability tests suggests it may be useful as a medical education resource. Nevertheless, more studies are required to assess the app's pedagogical effectiveness and make feature enhancements according to user input. Healthcare training and results will be enhanced as a result of the continuing efforts within the action design research methodology to optimize the app and advance its use in medical education. The potential of augmented reality to solve important educational problems in healthcare training is only going to increase as the technology develops further, opening up new possibilities for more efficient and accessible education.

REFERENCES

1. Lastrucci, Andrea, et al. "Exploring augmented reality integration in diagnostic imaging: myth or reality?" *Diagnostics* 14.13 (2024): 1333.
2. Amara, K., et al. "Augmented reality visualization and interaction for covid-19 ct-scan nn automated segmentation: a validation study." *IEEE Sensors Journal* 23.11 (2023): 12114–12123.

3. Goo, Hyun Woo, Sang Joon Park, and Shi-Joon Yoo. "Advanced medical use of three-dimensional imaging in congenital heart disease: augmented reality, mixed reality, virtual reality, and three-dimensional printing." *Korean Journal of Radiology* 21.2 (2020): 133–145.
4. González Izard, Santiago, et al. "Nextmed: automatic imaging segmentation, 3D reconstruction, and 3D model visualization platform using augmented and virtual reality." *Sensors* 20.10 (2020): 2962.
5. Venkatesan, Mythreye, Harini Mohan, Justin R. Ryan, Christian M. Schürch, Garry P. Nolan, David H. Frakes, and Ahmet F. Coskun. "Virtual and augmented reality for biomedical applications." *Cell Reports Medicine* 2.7 (2021).
6. Guerroudji, Mohamed Amine, et al. "A 3D visualization-based augmented reality application for brain tumor segmentation."
7. Kumar, T. Rajasanthosh, G. Laxmaiah, and S. Solomon Raj. "A Framework of Intelligent Manufacturing Process by Integrating Various Function." In Deepa Jose, Preethi Nanjundan, Sanchita Paul, and Sachi Nandan Mohanty (eds) *AI-Driven IoT Systems for Industry 4.0*, pp. 241–254. CRC Press, 2024.
8. Liu, Jiaqing, et al. "Augmented reality visualization and quantification of COVID-19 infections in the lungs." *Electronics* 13.6 (2024): 1158.
9. Patro, Pramoda, R. Azhagumurugan, R. Sathya, Krishna Kumar, T. Rajasanthosh Kumar, and M. Vijaya Sekhar Babu. "A hybrid approach estimates the real-time health state of a bearing by accelerated degradation tests, Machine learning." In *2021 Second International Conference on Smart Technologies in Computing, Electrical and Electronics (ICSTCEE)*, pp. 1–9. IEEE, 2021.
10. Rachmad, Yoesoep Edhie. *Augmented Health: The New Reality of Augmented Reality in Medical Practice*. Health Promotion Perspectives Publishing, Tabriz Book Special Issue, 2021.
11. Sahija, Dhaval. "Critical review of mixed reality integration with medical devices for patientcare." *International Journal for Innovative Research in Multidisciplinary Field* 8 (2022): 100–105.
12. Govinda Rajulu, G., M. Jamuna Rani, D. Deepa, Udit Mamodiya, Radhika G. Deshmukh, and T. Rajasanthosh Kumar. "Cloud-Computed Solar Tracking System." In Suresh Chandra Satapathy, Jerry Chun-Wei Lin, Lai Khin Wee, Vikrant Bhateja, T. M. Rajesh (eds) *Computer Communication, Networking and IoT: Proceedings of 5th ICICC 2021, Volume 2*, pp. 75–85. Singapore: Springer Nature Singapore, 2022
13. Moon, In Tae, et al. "Augmented reality in cardiology: enhancing visualization and precision." *Current Cardiovascular Risk Reports* 18.12 (2024): 175–186.
14. Rathore, P. S., S. Ahuja, S. R. Burri, A. Khunteta, A. Baliyan, & A. Kumar (2024). *Deep learning techniques for automation and industrial applications*. John Wiley & Sons, Inc.; Scrivener Publishing LLC.
15. Su, Mei-Ting, et al. "An acupoint health care system with real-time acupoint localization and visualization in augmented reality." *Multimedia Systems* 29.4 (2023): 2217–2238.
16. Kukla, Paulina, et al. "Extended reality in diagnostic imaging—a literature review." *Tomography* 9.3 (2023): 1071–1082.

17. Zhou, Kanglei, et al. "A video-based augmented reality system for human-in-the-loop muscle strength assessment of juvenile dermatomyositis." *IEEE Transactions on Visualization and Computer Graphics* 29.5 (2023): 2456–2466.
18. Haykal, Diala, Hugues Cartier, and Frederic Flament. "A Psychosocial Exploration of Augmented Reality and Virtual Reality Apps in Cosmetic Procedures." *Journal of Cosmetic Dermatology* 23.12 (2024): 3863–3870.
19. Taha, Bakr Ahmed, et al. "Photonics-powered augmented reality skin electronics for proactive healthcare: multifaceted opportunities." *Microchimica Acta* 191.5 (2024): 250.
20. Singh, Bhupinder, Komal Vig, and Christian Kaunert. "Modernizing healthcare: application of augmented reality and virtual reality in clinical practice and medical education." In Kamal Kant Hiran, et al. (eds) *Modern Technology in Healthcare and Medical Education: Blockchain, IoT, AR, and VR*. IGI Global, 2024. 1–21.
21. von Ende, Elizabeth, et al. "Artificial intelligence, augmented reality, and virtual reality advances and applications in interventional radiology." *Diagnostics* 13.5 (2023): 892.
22. Minopoulos, Georgios M., et al. "A medical image visualization technique assisted with AI-based haptic feedback for robotic surgery and healthcare." *Applied Sciences* 13.6 (2023): 3592.
23. Paul, Trishna, and Mukesh Kumar Rohil. "Utilization of Augmented Reality Visualizations in Healthcare Education: Trends and Future Scope." In *2023 IEEE Engineering Informatics*, Melbourne, Australia. pp. 1–10. IEEE, 2023.
24. Villagran-Vizcarra, Dafnis Cain, et al. "Applications analyses, challenges and development of augmented reality in education, industry, marketing, medicine, and entertainment." *Applied Sciences* 13.5 (2023): 2766.
25. Iqbal, Arham I., et al. "Immersive technologies in healthcare: an in-depth exploration of virtual reality and augmented reality in enhancing patient care, medical education, and training paradigms." *Journal of Primary Care & Community Health* 15 (2024): 21501319241293311.
26. Judy, Brendan F., et al. "Augmented reality and virtual reality in spine surgery: a comprehensive review." *Neurosurgery Clinics* 35.2 (2024): 207–216.

CHAPTER 12

Assessing Patient Outcomes in VR-Based Surgical Training

Kiran Kumar Maguluri, Zakera Yasmeen, Chandrashekar Pandugula, and Aaluri Seenu

12.1 INTRODUCTION

Minimally invasive surgery (MAS) and laparoscopic cholecystectomy have changed the way surgery is trained and accredited [1]. It became clear that the laparoscopy method was linked to a much higher rate of problems as MAS became more popular, especially when doctors were just starting to do these kinds of treatments [2, 3]. Although there were several factors at play, these advancements might be traced back to a lack of preparation for the psychomotor challenges presented by the visual interface [4]. As with other surgical training programs implemented over the last century, laparoscopic surgical education has mostly adhered to the tried-and-true mentor-trainee framework [5–8]. Surgical education institutions are on the lookout for cutting-edge training resources to keep up with the increasing complexity of modern surgical procedures as the new century begins [9–11].

Alongside MAS's expansion, other developments have drawn significant attention to the problem of medical mistakes [12]. The new and improved evidence-based training is required and possible has previously been acknowledged by surgeons, who were already aware of concerns such as the fact that improved training and objective evaluation could be crucial tactics for achieving the aim of fewer surgical mistakes [13–15].

DOI: 10.1201/9781003564904-12

Surgical skills training in VR was first suggested almost ten years ago, based on the effective model of flight simulation [16]. In addition to the improvement of desktop computers since then, useful and readily available VR-based surgery teachers and models have been created [17–20]. Surgeries have been practiced and graded using VR-based tools. According to the data, VR training is at least as equally effective as, if not more effective than, programs that use regular box trainers for learning basic skills [21–24]. VR training has not been shown to enhance surgeons' efficiency in an OR, which is the standard of excellence for any training approach [25–28]. However, no research has shown that VR training improves surgeons' performance in the OR [29, 30]. The research is conducted as part of the VR to OR program effort to find out whether the information learned about virtual reality in the skills lab transfers to the actual operating room. For this study, researcherd chose a typical laparoscopic surgery and a virtual reality trainer exercise that would help students learn the necessary skills for the operation.

12.2 METHODOLOGY

This research included 17 medical students from the surgical department in postgraduate category (PG), 11 of whom were male and 6 of whom were female. Every participant in the research was randomized to either the control group, which would get surgical training (ST) alone, or the study group, which would get the VR training in parallel with the conventional programmed training suitable for PG level. PG was used to classify the participants. To evaluate basic skills, every person in both groups took a set of previously approved assessments. The Cards Rotation, Cube Comparison, and Map Plan tasks were administered on pencil and paper as part of the visuospatial assessment [14]. Using the Graphical Surface Orientation exam (GicSOr), perceptual capacity (reorganization of three-dimensional pictures from two-dimensional pictures) was evaluated on a laptop computer. Using the Multimodal Invasive Surgical Trainer-VR (MIST VR) system, psychomotor competence was evaluated. All activities were placed at a medium degree of difficulty.

12.2.1 Devices

The MIST VR systems operated on a desktop computer (400-megahertz Pentium 2, 64-megabytes random-access memory), with tasks shown on a 17-inch CRT screen aligned with the operator's eye level. The video subsystem used (Matrox Mystique, eight-megabyte SD random-access memory)

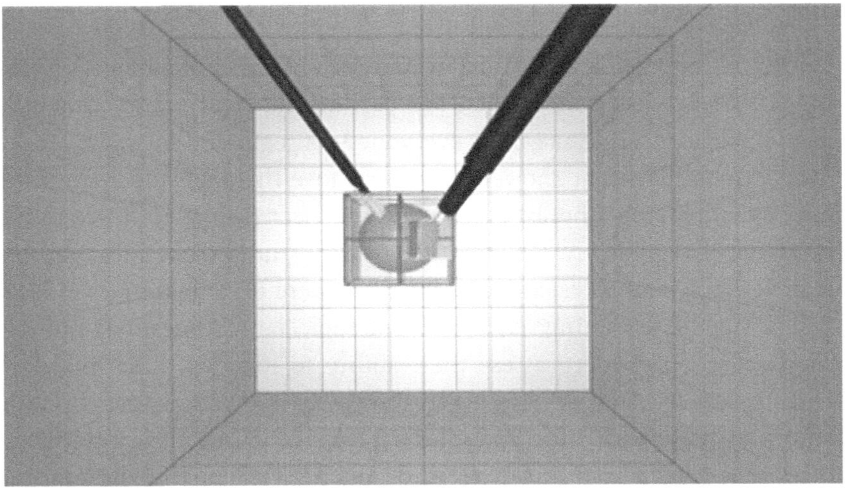

FIGURE 12.1 Schematic view of diathermy work in MIST VR.

achieved a frame rate of around 15 frames per second, enabling near–real-time translation of instrument motions to the visual display. Position-sensing gimbals with 6 degrees of freedom set two laparoscopic devices at an appropriate surgical height in relation to the operator in a frame, and a foot pedal for activating simulated electrosurgery tools made up the laparoscopy interface input system. This approach depicts an appropriately sized operational environment as a three-dimensional "box" on the computer display. Using virtual tools, targets may be gripped and moved about the working environment based on the particular skill challenge chosen (Figure 12.1). Every activity is documented as it is completed, allowing for precise and trustworthy evaluation.

12.2.2 Guidelines

Ten trials of the MIST VR "Manipulate and Diathermy" task were performed by five attending surgeons, all of whom had substantial previous expertise with laparoscopic operations at the "Tough" level to set performance criteria at mean economy of diathermy score 2 and mean error score 50. The objective of the virtual reality training session for the residents was to demonstrate equal proficiency with both hands on two separate trials at the levels established by the experienced specialized surgeons. The duration of each training session was about an hour. One of the authors monitored the training sessions at all times, and the authors paid close attention to minimizing errors and using as little diathermy as possible.

12.2.3 Techniques for Operations

One of the surgeon-investigators, who were blinded to the subject's training position, assisted all residents in performing laparoscopic cholecystectomy. Prior to the surgeries, everyone was requested to watch a brief instructional film that showed how to remove the gallbladder from the liver by employing a hook-type monopolar electrosurgical device in the most effective manner. The particular departures from ideal performance that would be regarded as mistakes were described in this video. Following the screening, each resident took a nine-question multiple choice test designed to assess their ability to identify these mistakes. During surgery, trainees are asked to cut out the gallbladder utilizing a normal two-handed method after carefully dividing the cystic structures that had been precisely located. During this part of the process, the attending surgeon communicated on video and radio, explaining any changes that were made (attending takeover of either of the tools). Procedures that involved a watching takeover were marked so that the audio could be reviewed.

12.2.4 Definition of Error

The five surgeon investigators along with a behavioral scientist working on the study watched old videotapes of laparoscopic cholecystectomy without any restrictions. They talked about possible ways to measure how successfully the surgery went. From the following listed definitions, eight events related to the cutting part of the process were noted as mistakes and used as study data.

- **No Progress**: During the whole minute of the surgery, no work was made on cutting out the liver. Dealing with the effects of a previously stated mistake is the same as not making progress if the gallbladder is not removed during this time.
- **Gallbladder Damage**: Gallbladder wall perforation may occur with or without bile leaking. Either hand is equally vulnerable to injury.
- **Liver Damage**: In addition to capsule stripping both with and without accompanying hemorrhage, there is liver capsules and parenchyma penetration.
- **Wrong Plane of Dissection**: The dissection is done in a plane that is not in the known plane among the gallbladder and the liver. It is done at the submucosal plane for the subcapsular plane for the liver.

- **Destroy Nontarget Tissue**: The use of electrocautery on nontarget tissues, with the possible exclusion of the latter portion of the fundic dissection, when present transmission may happen.
- **Soft Tissue Injury**: Tissues that are torn uncontrollably by the retracting or dissecting tool.
- **The Instrument Is Not Visible**: The cutting tool is used out of the telescope's field of view so that its tip can't be seen and could be touching cell material. A cutting tool going out of view because of a quick movement of the telescope will not be seen as a mistake.
- **Proceeding to the Takeover**: A portion of the surgery is carried out by the supervising attending surgeon using the resident's retracting tool (left hand) or dissecting instrument (right hand).

Any implications drawn from these measures that could not be seen directly were not included. For the purpose of promoting interrater agreement, each event was clearly specified. The criteria for determining whether an event was considered to have happened or not were clearly laid forth. Additionally, the duration of the gallbladder removal stage was determined. The duration of the surgery began when the electrosurgical device made its initial contact with tissue and finished when the gallbladder's last link to the liver was severed.

12.2.5 Evaluation of Interrater Compatibility

Two surgeon-investigators watched each procedural film silently, oblivious to the presence of any members of the surgical team. To keep track of whether errors happened during each 60-second interval, observers used a scoring matrix that allowed them to rate the gallbladder excision portion of the surgery minute-by-minute. Employing fixed-interval time-frame sampling, researchers kept track of the number of errors, where each mistake event was scored once, regardless of the number of times it happened inside the 1-minute period. After joining takeover events, participants were given scores depending on how they did on the reported videos. The solution below was used to find the interobserver agreement for interval assessments: $\frac{Agree}{Agree + disagree} * 100$.

The data is presented as the standard error of the mean (SEM). Three different statistical tests were used for comparison: analysis of variances

(ANOVA), Mann-Whitney, and chi-square. The significance threshold was set at $P < 0.06$.

12.3 RESULTS

Specifically, none of the first set of tests showed any significant changes among the VR and ST groups (Figure 12.2(a–c)).

Randomly assigned to the VR group, all of the residents met the performance standards within four to nine lessons. The process of separating the gall bladder in the liver bed was finished successfully by all patients in both groups. The accuracy of ranking trainees' surgical skills during video reviews ranged from 85% to 100%. Compared to the ST group, the VR-trained group completed dissections 30% faster, however this disparity did not reach statistically significant levels (Figure 12.3).

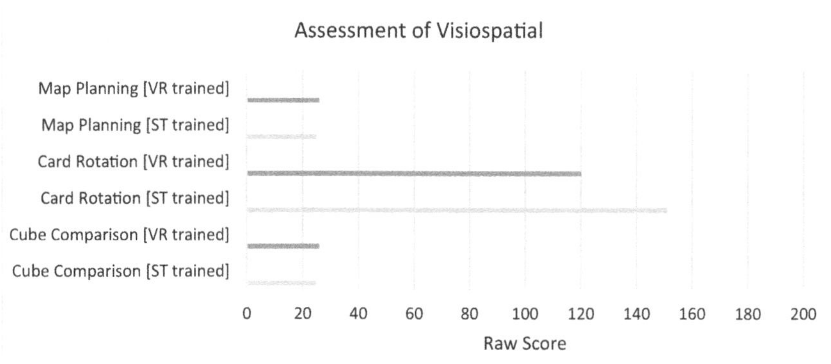

(a)

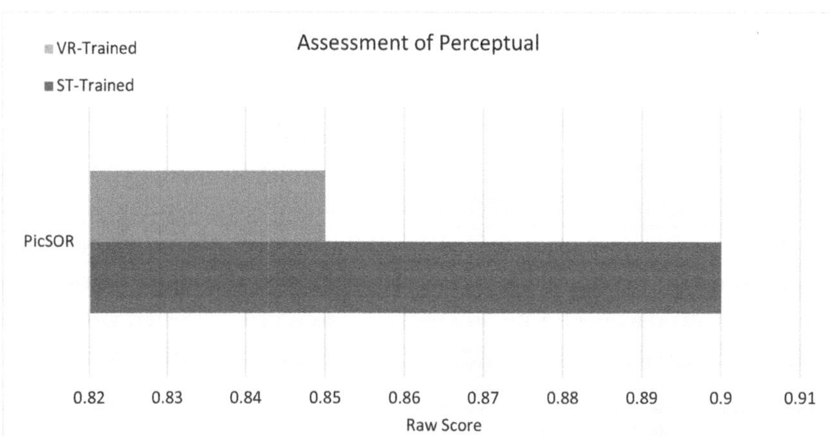

(b)

FIGURE 12.2 (a–c) Outcome of evaluation of basic skills.

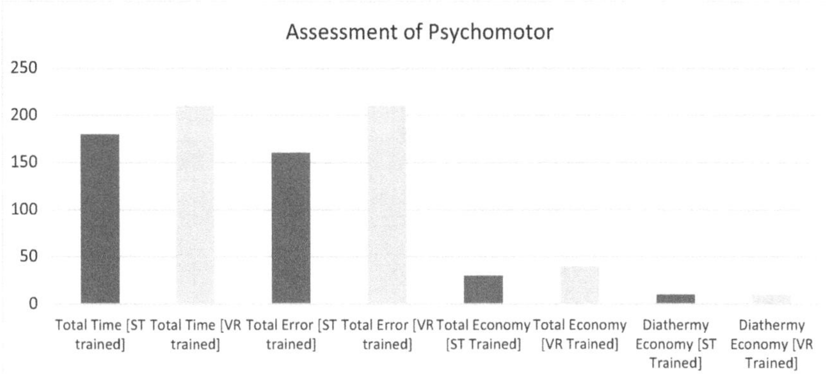

(c)

FIGURE 12.2 (Continued)

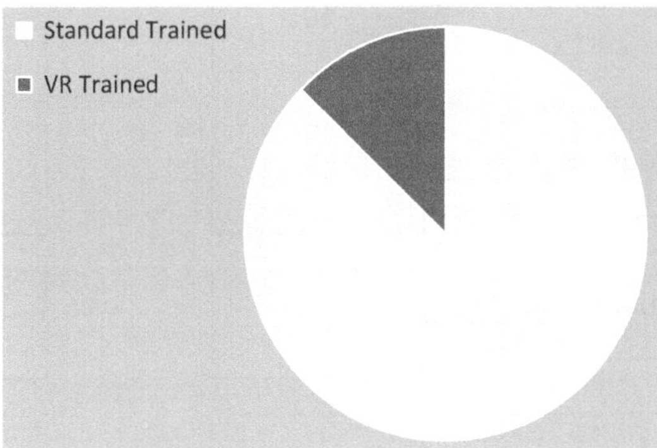

FIGURE 12.3 Average operative time period for ST and VR groups.

There was an increase of six in the risk of gallbladder damage along with burn of nontarget tissues mistakes in the ST group compared to the VR group. There was statistical significance in both instances when comparing each group for these mistakes separately [chi-squared test value is 4.28, $df = 1$, $P > 0.5$]. ST participants had a mean of 0.26 lack of progress mistakes per case, which is ten times higher than the 2.20 errors per case for non-ST residents. Not a single mistake was made with breaking tissue in either group. One damage to the liver, three wrong incision planes, and six mistakes made by the assisting surgeon during takeover were all found among the ST category. More mistakes were made in the ST category compared with the VR category in every category except liver damage (one mistake in the VR category) and tearing tissues (nil mistakes in either category) (Figure 12.4).

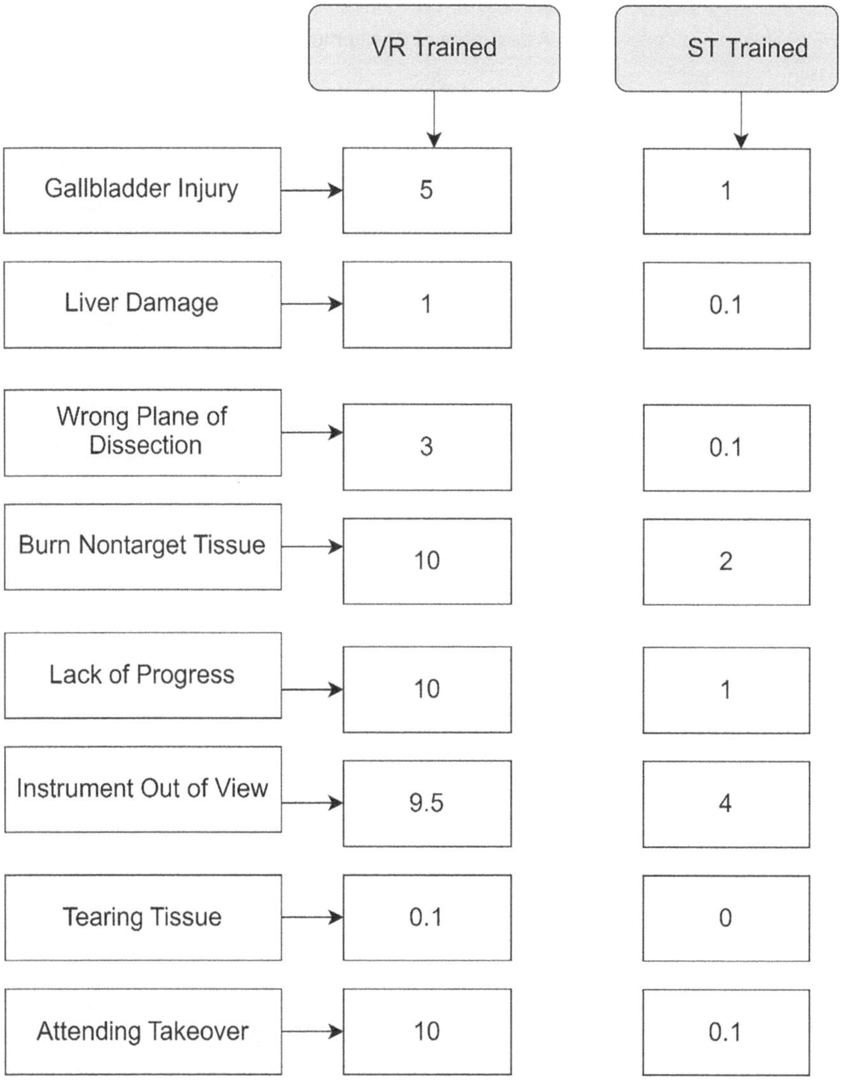

FIGURE 12.4 Types of errors occurred in VR and ST groups.

Standard errors showed that the VR residents' performance varied five times as much as the ST group, resulting in nearly seven times the errors than the VR team (Figure 12.5). Compared to the VR group, the ST group had a considerably higher mean number of assessed mistakes for each operation.

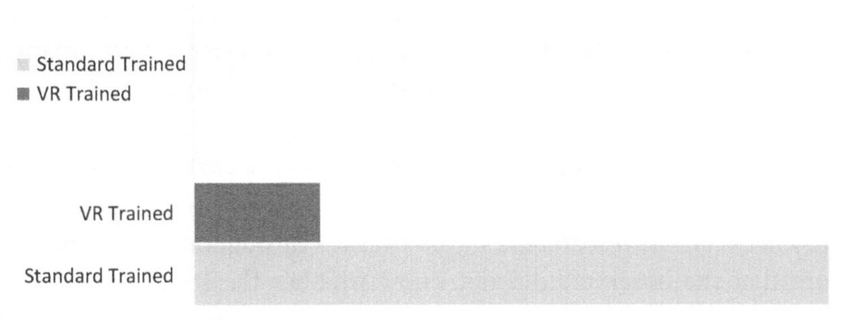

FIGURE 12.5 Error count for each operation in the VR and ST groups.

12.4 DISCUSSION

The study's findings show that even surgical trainees without a lot of previous surgical experience may benefit from virtual reality training for operating skills. Less mistakes were made, there was a lower chance of gallbladder damage and nontarget tissue burning, and residents who received MIST VR training were more likely to move steadily through the process. Residents were informed throughout VR training that speed wasn't a key training factor. Instead, instruction focused on placing "tissue" with the non-dissecting hand and using electrosurgery tools safely and economically. Skilled laparoscopic surgeons predetermined certain objective performance criteria to be met in order to complete the training process. Though it was unclear throughout research planning if these criteria levels were excessive, pilot testing proved that residents were able to accomplish them. This is a crucial consideration, as setting the standard too high could make it unattainable for the participants in the study. The VR-trained group showed consistent performance in the OR phase of the trial, which may have been due in part to these targeted performance levels. Because the resident had to meet clear performance standards on two straight tries, it was rare that they would do so by accident. The laparoscopic doctors set a performance standard level that needs to be confirmed by the rest of the medical community to see if these are the right numbers and levels to show "expert" performance.

It is necessary to establish the link between laboratory assessment and training methodologies and OR performance, irrespective of how advanced they become. Measurement of observable surgical performance was the goal of our operational evaluation methodology. No conclusions were made on the reason behind the resident's specific performance. Instead of using Likert-type scales or global assessments of resident performance, a fixed-interval time frame sampling technique was used to determine whether or not predetermined mistake occurrences were present. Because the focus was on events that could be seen, the level of dependability between the researchers stayed over 0.9 throughout the study. This meant that the observers did not know whether the study participants were trained or not. Similar mistakes have been examined in the past when trying to figure out how well laparoscopic cholecystectomy works, but they reviewed the whole operation. This method was clearly possible and dependable, but it took a lot of time at the training and marking stages.

The focus of this study is on a straightforward operational assignment that places a priority on technical abilities. "Errors" in surgical technique were characterized as isolated occurrences that deviated significantly from ideal performance without associating these occurrences with negative consequences or direct causes. These mistakes were tracked and assessed, which made it possible to evaluate how well VR training worked to lower their frequency. The achievement of this research goal was made possible by the operational procedure's simplicity. Nevertheless, competence includes a variety of physical and cognitive abilities that are not always amenable to standardized assessment. More advanced techniques for identifying and evaluating certain abilities at the OR remain necessary given that VR training is expected to quickly become more diverse and realistic. In order to eradicate practices that result in unfavourable clinical results, researchers foresee applying similar training techniques to additional procedures.

Significant progress has been made in surgical education with the confirmation of virtual reality training's efficacy in improving operating abilities. Prior to operating on a patient, a resident may be required to demonstrate a high degree of objectively evaluated competence. One benefit of VR trainers and simulators is that they may accommodate as much or as little training as is necessary to get the desired objective. An investigator oversaw and guided the residents through training activities to ensure the system's validity in our research. As of right now, surgical students may practice anytime they choose, and the simulator will keep checking their proficiency until they reach competency. Mentoring the training work on a computer is also viable with the right tools. Technical skills will soon be able to be "trained out" on a simulator instead of on real patients. This means that students may receive significant amounts of help without taking up too much of their supervisor's time. Every time someone uses a VR simulator, their performance is recorded and logged. This gives the program director an automatic quality control tool for judging how effectively someone is improving their basic technical skills. There are many other skills that a surgeon learns in addition to the ones they practice on the simulators. These include cognitive skills like recognizing anatomy, figuring out alternate plans, and more. The research, on the other hand, established for the very first time that VR training has a significant role in improving the capability of surgical students to carry out an operation with a more effective and, one might argue, safer performance. It is for this reason that our results provide support to the incorporation of virtual reality practice into surgical educational initiatives.

12.5 CONCLUSION

Virtual reality training has the potential to lower the frequency of intraoperative mistakes and problems, which is one of its main advantages. Researchers have shown that surgeons who practice on virtual reality simulators are more capable to handle anatomical differences and avoid dangerous areas like the bile duct and large blood vessels during real surgeries. This has the potential to reduce the occurrence of surgical problems such as bleeding, perforation of nearby organs, and injury to the bile ducts. Additionally, unlike with conventional clinical training, virtual reality simulations may help surgeons be prepared for those unusual but possibly fatal cases. The end result is an increase in patient safety due to improved preparation and faster decision-making.

Virtual reality–based surgical training shows promise for boosting patient outcomes for cholecystectomy, or gallbladder removal. Surgeons may train and improve their abilities in a secure and monitored setting using VR, which improves their technical competency and decision-making. Research shows that when used in clinical practice, virtual reality training may result in better surgical performance, reduced mistake rates, and quicker procedure times. A better comprehension of intricate processes is also promoted by VR's ability to simulate scenarios and provide additional training. VR's incorporation in medical education is probably going to keep improving surgical proficiency and, eventually, patient safety and recovery as the technology develops.

A considerable improvement in the overall performance of residents in the operating room during laparoscopic cholecystectomy was achieved with the use of virtual reality surgical simulation to meet particular requirements. As a result of this confirmation of the transfer of training abilities from virtual reality to the operating room, the foundation has been laid for more advanced applications of VR in the assessment, training, minimization of errors, and licensing of surgeons.

VR gallbladder removal training has provided promising surgical success; however, it faces significant obstacles to general adoption. Low-resource medical institutions may not be able to afford high-quality VR simulators. VR training platforms work effectively when the simulation is realistic and mimics real-life surgical situations. Standards and clinical relevance of VR simulation techniques must be maintained. Experienced doctors may be hesitant of VR-based teaching, particularly if they prefer hands-on mentoring. Proof of advantages and ongoing professional growth are needed to close this disparity.

REFERENCES

1. Gallagher, Anthony G., et al. "Virtual reality simulation for the operating room: proficiency-based training as a paradigm shift in surgical skills training." *Annals of Surgery* 241.2 (2005): 364–372.
2. Aydin, Abdullatif, et al. "Simulation-based training and assessment in urological surgery." *Nature Reviews Urology* 13.9 (2016): 503–519.
3. Shaharan, Shazrinizam, and Paul Neary. "Evaluation of surgical training in the era of simulation." *World Journal of Gastrointestinal Endoscopy* 6.9 (2014): 436.
4. Pfandler, Michael, et al. "Virtual reality-based simulators for spine surgery: a systematic review." *The Spine Journal* 17.9 (2017): 1352–1363.
5. Thomsen, Ann Sofia Skou, et al. "Operating room performance improves after proficiency-based virtual reality cataract surgery training." *Ophthalmology* 124.4 (2017): 524–531.
6. Vaughan, Neil, et al. "A review of virtual reality based training simulators for orthopaedic surgery." *Medical Engineering & Physics* 38.2 (2016): 59–71.
7. Dhotre, Virendrakumar Anna, Habibulla Mohammad, Prakash Kumar Pathak, Anurag Shrivastava, and T. Rajasanthosh Kumar. "Big data analytics using MapReduce for education system." *Linguistica Antverpiensia* (2021): 3130–3138.
8. Hong, Minsik, Jerzy W. Rozenblit, and Allan J. Hamilton. "Simulation-based surgical training systems in laparoscopic surgery: a current review." *Virtual Reality* 25.2 (2021): 491–510.
9. Alaker, Medhat, Greg R. Wynn, and Tan Arulampalam. "Virtual reality training in laparoscopic surgery: a systematic review & meta-analysis." *International Journal of Surgery* 29 (2016): 85–94.
10. Larsen, Christian R., et al. "Effect of virtual reality training on laparoscopic surgery: randomised controlled trial." *BMJ* 338 (2009): b1802.

11. Aydın, Abdullatif, et al. "Effect of simulation-based training on surgical proficiency and patient outcomes: a randomised controlled clinical and educational trial." *European Urology* 81.4 (2022): 385–393.
12. Kumar, T. Rajasanthosh, Kesaraju Venkata Sai Pavan, Rajesh Kukati, and Mandala Srinivasa Reddy. "Quantitatively examines the feasibility of different configurations of the aftermarket supply chain enabling additive manufacturing." *Solid State Technology* 63.5 (2020): 492–507.
13. Lawaetz, Jonathan, et al. "Simulation based training and assessment in open vascular surgery: a systematic review." *European Journal of Vascular and Endovascular Surgery* 61.3 (2021): 502–509.
14. Moglia, Andrea, et al. "A systematic review of virtual reality simulators for robot-assisted surgery." *European Urology* 69.6 (2016): 1065–1080.
15. Seymour, Neal E., et al. "Virtual reality training improves operating room performance: results of a randomized, double-blinded study." *Annals of Surgery* 236.4 (2002): 458–464.
16. Dawe, Susan R., et al. "Systematic review of skills transfer after surgical simulation-based training." *Journal of British Surgery* 101.9 (2014): 1063–1076.
17. Zendejas, Benjamin, et al. "State of the evidence on simulation-based training for laparoscopic surgery: a systematic review." *Annals of Surgery* 257.4 (2013): 586–593.
18. Beyer-Berjot, Laura, et al. "Surgical training: design of a virtual care pathway approach." *Surgery* 156.3 (2014): 689–697.
19. Aïm, Florence, et al. "Effectiveness of virtual reality training in orthopaedic surgery." *Arthroscopy: The Journal of Arthroscopic & Related Surgery* 32.1 (2016): 224–232.
20. Aggarwal, Rajesh, et al. "Proving the effectiveness of virtual reality simulation for training in laparoscopic surgery." *Annals of Surgery* 246.5 (2007): 771–779.
21. Pulijala, Yeshwanth, et al. "Effectiveness of immersive virtual reality in surgical training—a randomized control trial." *Journal of Oral and Maxillofacial Surgery* 76.5 (2018): 1065–1072.
22. Sturm, Lana P., et al. "A systematic review of skills transfer after surgical simulation training." *Annals of Surgery* 248.2 (2008): 166–179.
23. Shahrezaei, Aidin, et al. "The impact of surgical simulation and training technologies on general surgery education." *BMC Medical Education* 24.1 (2024): 1297.
24. van der Meijden, Olivier A. J., and Marlies P. Schijven. "The value of haptic feedback in conventional and robot-assisted minimal invasive surgery and virtual reality training: a current review." *Surgical Endoscopy* 23 (2009): 1180–1190.
25. Lee, Jason Y., et al. "Validation study of a virtual reality robotic simulator—role as an assessment tool?." *The Journal of Urology* 187.3 (2012): 998–1002.
26. Bruppacher, Heinz R., et al. "Simulation-based training improves physicians' performance in patient care in high-stakes clinical setting of cardiac surgery." *The Journal of the American Society of Anesthesiologists* 112.4 (2010): 985–992.

27. Cosman, Peter H., et al. "Virtual reality simulators: current status in acquisition and assessment of surgical skills." *ANZ Journal of Surgery* 72.1 (2002): 30–34.
28. Chan, Justin, et al. "A systematic review of virtual reality for the assessment of technical skills in neurosurgery." *Neurosurgical Focus* 51.2 (2021): E15.
29. Zendejas, Benjamin, et al. "Simulation-based mastery learning improves patient outcomes in laparoscopic inguinal hernia repair: a randomized controlled trial." *Annals of Surgery* 254.3 (2011): 502–511.
30. Lee, Gyusung I., and Mija R. Lee. "Can a virtual reality surgical simulation training provide a self-driven and mentor-free skills learning? Investigation of the practical influence of the performance metrics from the virtual reality robotic surgery simulator on the skill learning and associated cognitive workloads." *Surgical Endoscopy* 32 (2018): 62–72.

CHAPTER 13

Optimizing Practical Training for First Responders Using VR

Gowtham Mandala, Breeze Tripathi, and R. Senthamil Selvan

13.1 INTRODUCTION

Radiology is becoming increasingly important in medical evaluation. Radiology tests, like computed tomography (CT), are very important in today's healthcare because healthcare professionals can't always tell what's wrong with a person just by looking at them [1]. Recent national trends show increased use of CT scans. The total cost of medical imaging is thought to have gone up from about US$101 billion to about $201 billion dollars today. Imaging prices for women using Medicare was $518 per person. How can we lower these rising costs? This is a very important question [2–5]. Researchers believe that mixing augmented reality (AR) and virtual reality (VR) with 3D medical scans could help find some answers. It is the goal of this study to explore the integration of imaging technologies and demonstrate their potential benefits. This chapter consists of three parts [6–15]. First, it discusses cross-sectional imaging and how it works, focusing on CT and MRI scans and their limitations. Next, it explores advancements in visualization techniques such as surface rendering, volume rendering, and depth-three-dimensional (D3D) imagery that combines AR and VR imaging. The chapter then examines the current role AR plays in diagnostic medical images and some of the problems

DOI: 10.1201/9781003564904-13

that AR has helped solve. Finally, it looks ahead to the future potential of AR for accurate medical imaging [16–20].

13.1.1 Background on X-rays for Diagnostic Purposes

Diagnostic imaging has become more advanced thanks to advances in technology, but these changes have also brought new challenges for the radiologist. The researcher will take a quick look at the science behind CT and MRI in this section.

13.1.1.1 Computed Tomography

For CT scans, the patient lies flat on a motorized table that moves through a donut-shaped scanner. Inside the scanner, an X-ray tube along with an X-ray monitor rotate around the patient. As the X-ray detector unit moves around the patient, it takes several projection pictures. Through processing methods such as filtered back projection, this data is reconstructed into axial plane pictures again. After the axial plane images are reconstructed, the coronal and sagittal plane views are generated. An axial image's grid resolution is typically 513 × 513 pixels. Each pixel in the axial plane represents a flat 2D body with defined dimensions in the x- and y-directions. A Hounsfeld Unit (HU) is a grayscale value that is assigned to each pixel in a CT scan picture. This value depends on the type of tissue and how dense it is. Including the third dimension (z-direction) to an orthogonal pixel plane to make volume is one way to turn a pixel into a 3D shape, such as a cube [21]. For context, very dense materials, like compact bone, have an HU of about +1000 and very light things, like air, have an HU of −1000. The HU of water is 0. The brain, liver, kidneys, muscles, and other soft parts in the body have HUs that are about 41, slightly higher than water. With an HU of −101, fat is less dense than water (see Figure 13.1). Modern CT scans can now be performed quickly. For example, a full-body scan can be completed in 16 seconds with a precision of less than 2 mm. This has great potential for diagnosing diseases and assessing traumas. In trauma centres, "pan CT scans" from head to toe are valuable for looking at the inside of the body. By acting swiftly, the trauma surgeon can potentially save many patients.

13.1.1.2 Magnetic Resonance Imaging

For an MRI scan, the patient lies flat upon a scanning table, which is surrounded by a large, cylinder-shaped machine. A strong magnetic field is used in the MRI, and it is directed along the long line of the cylinder.

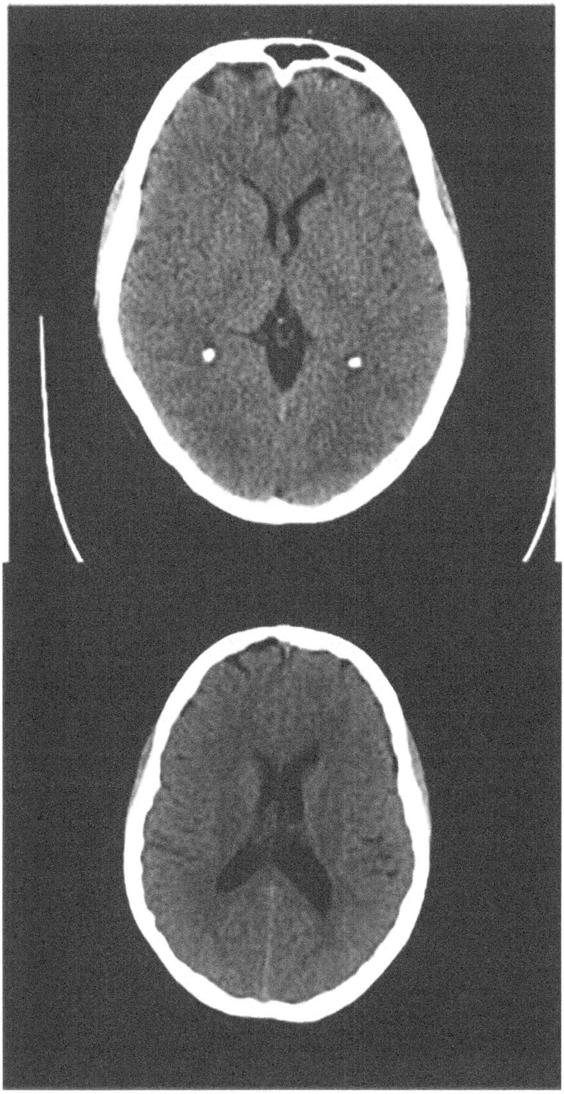

FIGURE 13.1 Axial plane images of a typical brain.
The head CT image (Top) displays the dense skull in white, the brain tissue in a medium gray hue, and cerebrospinal fluid in dark gray. The T2-weighted MRI picture (Bottom) depicts the skull in black, the brain in medium gray with superior contrast between gray matter and white matter, and cerebrospinal fluid in white.

Radiofrequency (RF) pulses are sent into the patient by transmitter coils and an image is made from the electromagnetic signal that comes back from the body by receiver coils. The main advantage of an MRI scan over a CT scan is that it can distinguish between different body tissues that have the same density. Additionally, MRI does not use ionizing radiation. This is possible with an MRI because different body tissues (brain cells, water, fat, iron, for example) react to magnetic fields in different ways. As an example, different types of tissues have different relaxation times when exposed to the radiofrequency (RF) stimulus [22–25]. This means that the MRI images offer varying signal strengths and excellent contrast between tissue types. MRI scans can be adjusted to differentiate between tissues that are densely packed together, such as the brain's gray matter and white matter. The blood vessels can be seen best with other specialized MRI scans. Like CT images, MRI images are composed of a grid, with each pixel assigned a numerical value corresponding to a specific shade of gray. Currently, getting an MRI scan takes much longer than getting a CT scan. For example, a brain MRI usually takes around two hours. However, MRI has better contrast clarity of some soft tissues, such as gray and white brain matter (Figure 13.1). This means that it can be used to make diagnoses that CT scans cannot.

13.1.1.3 Common Ways of Viewing Things and the Problems that Come with Them

Radiologists are struggling to keep up with all the new information because CT and MRI images now have much better spatial detail (often less than 2 mm). In the case of a chest CT, there are more than 501 sagittal plane images. Each slice may contain 513 × 513 pixels in each the x- and y-directions. The dataset would have 132 million images with 501 axial slices (z-direction). The gray shade at every location in the body is different and shows how dense the tissue is there. These differences are displayed on a standard 2D screen. In addition to axial plane images, radiologists also examine coronal and sagittal plane views. For a single chest CT test, this can add up to over 1001 images. It can be very hard for the radiologist to visually develop a 3D volume model for each 2D slice, given the complexity of human anatomy. Another problem that doctors have to deal with is ensuring that every point is carefully reviewed, which is especially critical for early cancer detection. Early cancer detection is crucial for two reasons: the survival of patients and the reduction of healthcare expenses.

However, in their early stages, tumours may be as small as a few pixels across and hardly noticeable compared to the surrounding tissue, with a range of grayscale tones. Their consequences may be quite harmful to patients, and they are easy to miss, often showing up for the first time in a very advanced state of cancer. It takes a long time to carefully look at something slice by slice. Because of the large, complex collections, new ways to review them have come up. In this study, we will talk about imaging methods that can help us see the complex 3D design of the human body better.

13.2 NEW DEVELOPMENTS IN VIEWING METHODS

13.2.1 Rendering the Surface

Surface modeling, also called colored surface projection, was one of the earliest techniques for visualizing the 3D structure of the human body. In this approach, segmentation methods, such as thresholding to isolate specific sets of pixels, are used to represent the body's visible surfaces. A virtual light source is then applied to shade the surface. Because only one area is chosen, this method isn't restricted by overlapping anatomical structures. There are some problems with surface modeling, though, because it can only show a small amount of information at a time. Additionally, many internal body's systems don't have clearly defined surfaces, making them difficult to render accurately. Also, although surface rendering pictures appear three dimensional due to shading, they do not provide true depth perception.

13.2.2 Rendering of Volume

Volume rendering is method that has long been studied in the fields of computer graphics and visualization, but has only recently been applied to diagnostic medical imaging. Unlike surface rendering, volume rendering doesn't usually need segmentation. But if segmentation is done during volume rendering, either the whole volume or a part of it can be kept. Usually, a transfer function is used to describe values of interest by giving each intensity value a colour and an opacity. This method needs more processing power than surface drawing, but it has some benefits. The main advantage is that it lets the doctor see the entire dataset at once. For example, it becomes much easier to understand how features in slice N relate to slice N+2. When 3D modelling is performed, image slices are stacked in the right order to make a volume of non-overlapping voxels.

It's much easier to keep track of over- and underlays when looking at volume output than when looking at it by individual slice. This has made it much easier for doctors to see complicated 3D structures like blood vessels. Applying a virtual light source, moving the volume (up and down and clockwise and counterclockwise), and zooming in and out are all tools used in volume modelling and AR/VR applications. Crossover is one of the main problems with volume modelling, as you can see in both Figures 13.2 and 13.3.

Several straight lines are drawn through the 3D space to the 2D image during this step. By showing the voxel in the ray with the highest level of light (or Hounsfield Units in CT), the maximum intensity projection (MIP) picture is made. Keep in mind that 2D imagery only shows light gray pixels, but the 3D volume has both dark gray as well as light gray voxels.

As you can see from the lines and ovals, there are several places where blood vessels meet. No matter what direction the volume rendering image

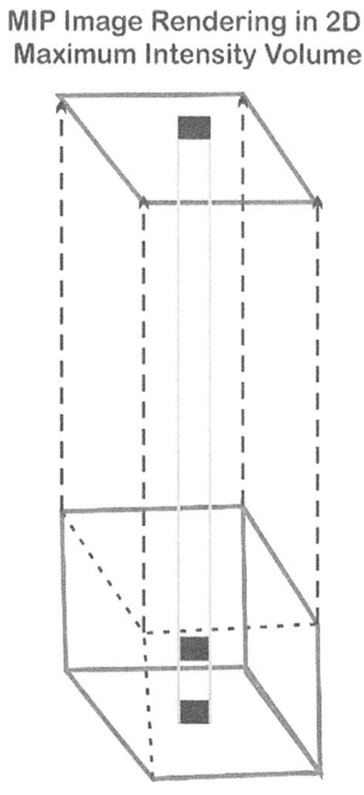

FIGURE 13.2 Volume drawing operates under maximum intensity projection (a MIP).

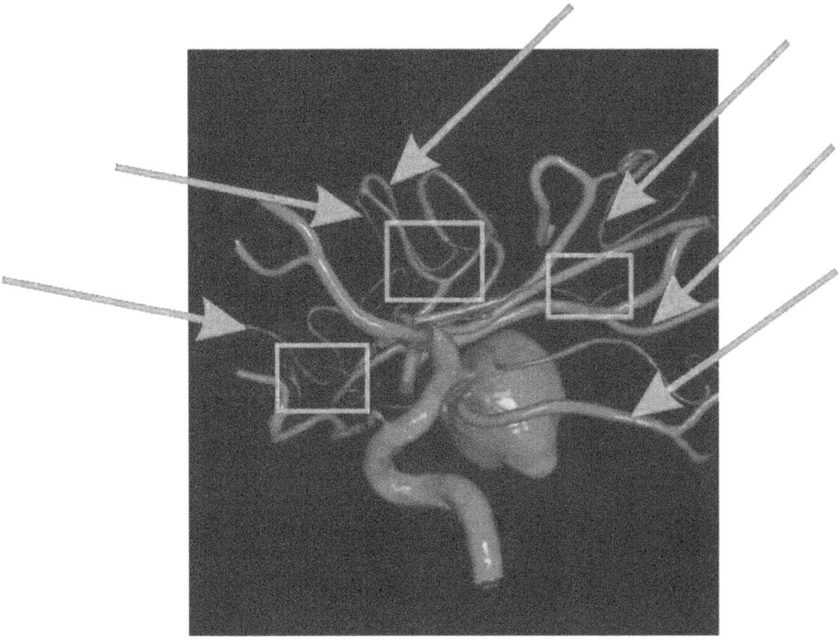

FIGURE 13.3 Volume representation of magnetic resonance angiography (or MRA) depicts the cerebral vasculature without other tissues.

is rotated, overlapping or intersecting vessels can remain visible, which makes interpretation harder. Because the images are computer-generated, elements such as artificial lighting and shadows are added, which could lead to misinterpretation.

Fishman et al. along with Johnson et al. both found that volume modelling can help show some complex anatomical structures, but they also said that it can be limited by anatomy that overlaps. A lot of work has gone into getting around this problem, such as importance-driven volume modelling, smart exposure, and curved planar rearrangement. "This is like examining a bowl of spaghetti," said one doctor, who preferred to use normal axial, sagittal, and coronal plane images rather than volume rendering images when interpreting the images. Many doctors have come to the conclusion that overlapping anatomical structures in volume-rendered images are difficult to interpret and cause concern thatthey might be missing something hidden behind other structures. High-definition computer monitors are common viewing screens for traditional volume modelling.

13.2.3 Imaging in Three Dimensions (D3D) with Depth

A user's choice of a head-mounted display (HMD) determines whether D3D is best suited for virtual reality or augmented reality. D3D users wear a binocular HMD which shows a different picture to each eye. This gives the user depth perception and visual differentiation. The different right and left viewing angles are made in real time based on what the user types into an extremely complex image processing algorithm. This algorithm works by focusing light on a single point, which is how light naturally enters the eye (see Figure 13.4). In addition to the 3D modelling, this method includes a unique context-based division and priority-based screening.

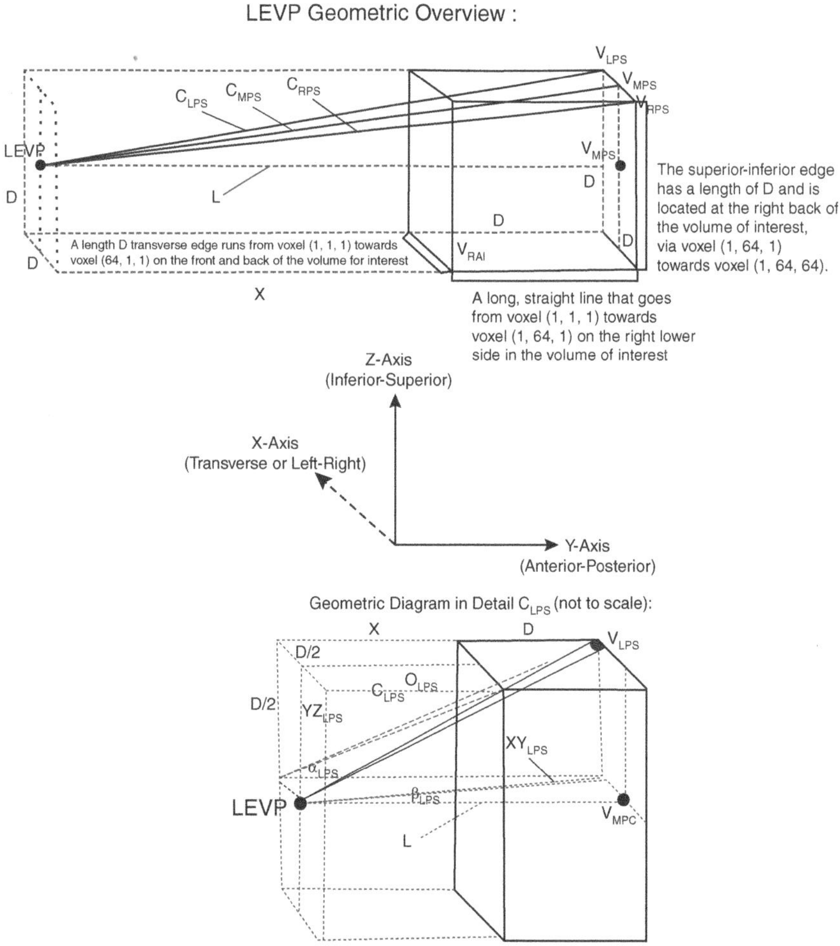

FIGURE 13.4 A left-eye D3D processing system overview.

13.2.4 Virtual Reality

In terms of VR technology, desktop computers are examples of non-intensive VR. Other types include semi-immersive and fully immersive VR. As with the Oculus Rift and HTC Vive, fully realistic VR fills the user's field of view with a simulated picture and blocks out all of the real world. When you use Samsung Gear VR, the HMD shows you a virtual image and blocks out some of the real world. This is an example of semi-immersive VR. The VR user can navigate by moving their head (tracked through the HMD) or by walking around (through external camera tracking). They can also use hand-held controllers with physical input or voice commands to interact with the virtual world. One problem with VR is difficulty in keeping the head steady, which can lead to motion sickness or discomfort.

The FDA (Food and Drug Administration) does not yet allow viewing medical images in virtual reality. One potential medical use of VR equipment is the imaging of breast cancer, one of the leading causes of death for women. It is important to identify whether the microcalcifications are "cluster," "linear," or "branching" in order to help assess the likelihood of cancer. The "branching" pattern is the most concerning for malignancy. A recent study used simulated breast microcalcification data and found that the D3D VR system was better at showing the linear and branching patterns of the microcalcifications than a flat screen. In fact, doctors misinterpreted the linear and branching patterns as clusters on the 2D monitor as a cluster, leading to false negatives. However, the D3D system correctly identified it as linear as well as branching, resulting in a true positive diagnosis. The study also noted that the HMD display and the joystick control system provided a more intuitive human–machine interface (HMI) via a more engaging fly-through experience that could rotate and zoom (see Figures 13.5 and 13.6).

Technologies that use augmented reality can be divided into two groups: AR and mixed reality (MR). Within both AR and MR, a virtual image as well as a real-world image are shown simultaneously. This lets the user communicate with both the real and virtual environments at the same time. In both technologies, the user wears an HMD that overlays digital content onto the real world. In AR, the virtual image appears semi-transparent, like a hologram, as seen in Meta and DAQRI systems. In contrast, the MR virtual content observed in the Microsoft HoloLens appears more solid and realistic.

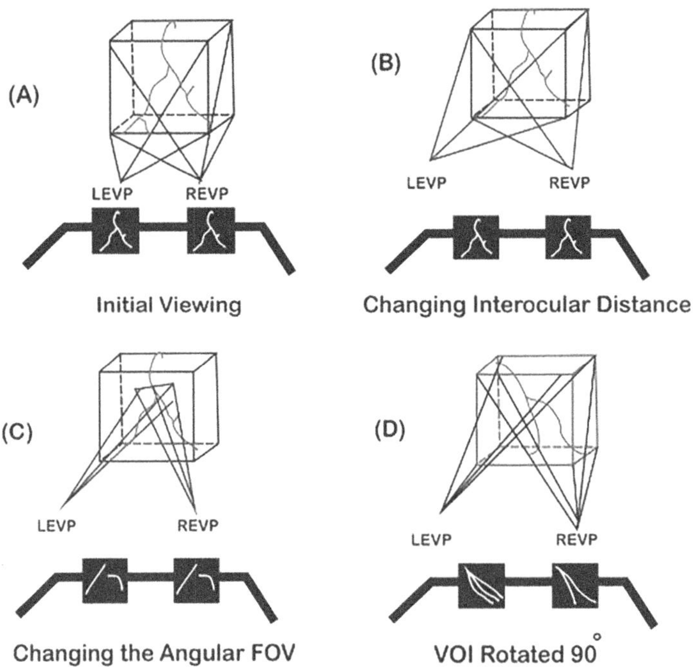

FIGURE 13.5 VR can be used with D3D.
With left eye view perspective (LEVP) as well as right eye viewing perspective (REVP), this image shows the head mounted display in gray goggles and a synthetic collection ofbreast microcalcifications. Note how D3D systems enhance the visualization ofmicrocalcifications: (A) the original viewinging angle; (B) decreasing the interocular distance to improve depth perception; (C) adjusting the field of view (FOV); and (D) rotating the volume of interest (VOI).

The FDA has not yet approved the medical use of AR displays for diagnostic imaging. The real-world image that AR is layered onto changes depending on the clinical task. In real life, the image would be the patient's body if a physical test and medical imagery review were done together, either before or during a surgical procedure. In other situations, the real-world image might show an operation room, a classroom, a reading room for X-rays, or a doctor's office.

13.2.4.1 The Use of AR in Breast Cancer Imaging for Diagnosis

In breast cancer detection, the radiologist's most important job is to correctly describe the mass's shape and edges to figure out how likely it is to be cancerous. Imaging is now an important part of treating breast cancer because it is known that tumour shrinking is linked to the efficiency of

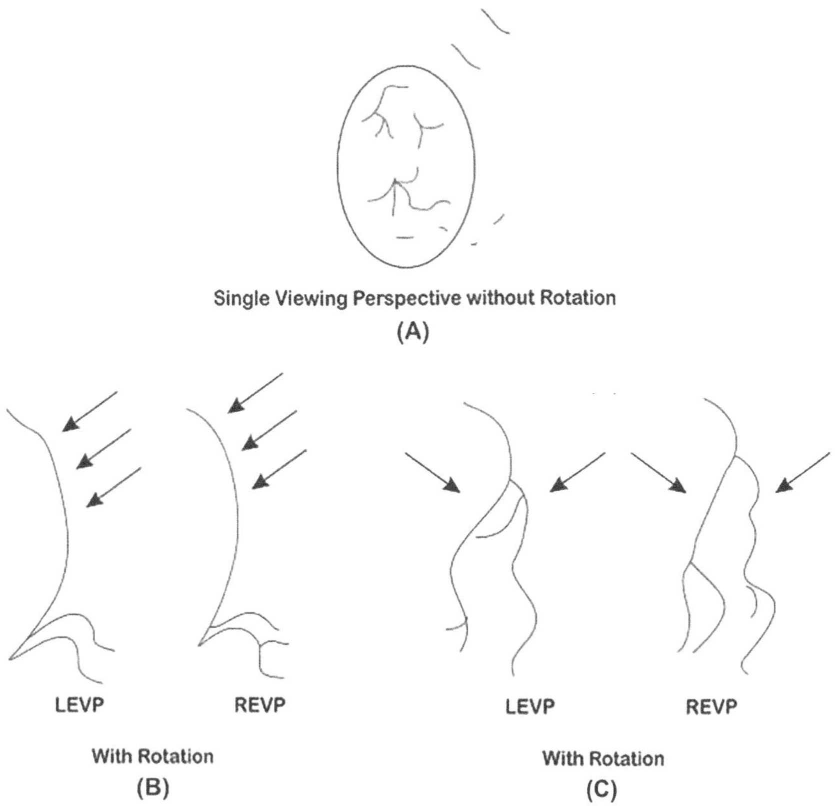

FIGURE 13.6 Images of simulated microcalcifications on the breast. (A) Shows how the virtual breast microcalcifications can be seen as a cluster with a single projection while (B) shows how identical breast microcalcifications can be seen with rotation on the VR D3D system. For reference, there are two images provided. One shows the LEVP and the other from the REVP. Keep in mind that this shows a straight line, which is a potential indicator of ductal carcinoma in situ (DCIS), a type of breast cancer. Image (C) demonstrates how similar breast microcalcifications can be visualized in 3D with the D3D system. The presence of linear and branching patterns is especially concerning for DCIS. In this case, the system correctly identified it as a true positive.

neoadjuvant chemotherapy (the NACT) in treating advanced breast cancer. The latest Investigation of Serial Studies to Predict Your Therapeutic Response with Imaging and moLecular Analysis 2 research showed that the shape of the breast tumour was important because the way the tumour borders appeared was linked to how well NACT worked. The shape of the growth also played a part in the doctor's decision about whether or not the patient would have breast conservation surgery or a mastectomy.

What MRI showed was a better indicator of disease reaction than a clinical exam. Dedicated breast CT images also show breast lumps with great detail, so the form and edges can be carefully examined. Spiculations, which are spike-like projections extending from the mass's surface, are a strong indicator of breast cancer. In one case, a known breast cancer was examined using a dedicated breast CT was evaluated with the D3D method. The physician reported that the shape, edges and spiculations of the mass were more easily visualized using the D3D method than with conventional 2D imaging (see Figure 13.7).

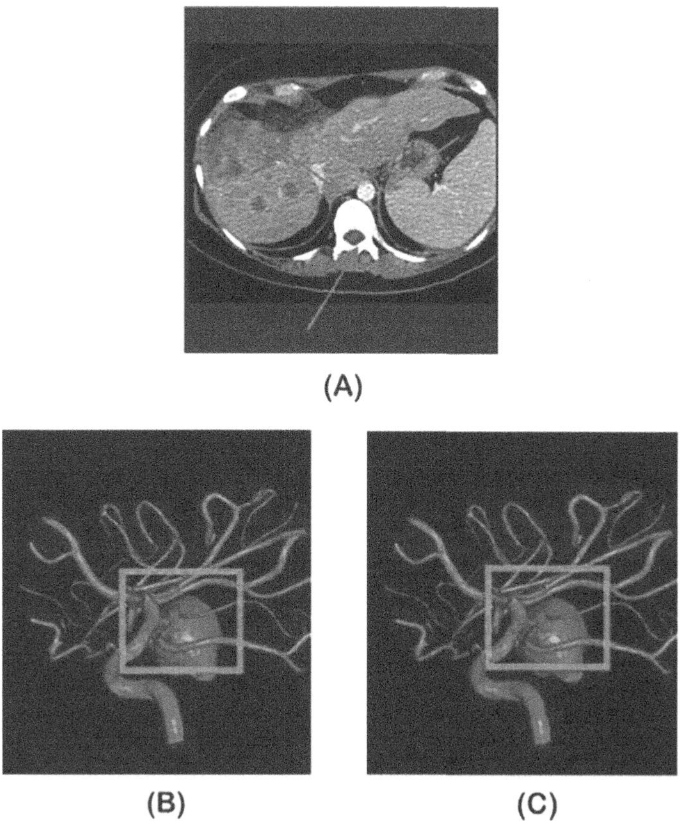

FIGURE 13.7 CT scans of a breast that has been diagnosed with cancer.
(A) Shows an axial CT scan of the breast mass, with the arrow pointing to spiculations at the edges of the tumour; (B and C) show LEVP along with REVP observed in D3D. Breast cancer is shown by the gray mass that surrounds the 3D cursor.

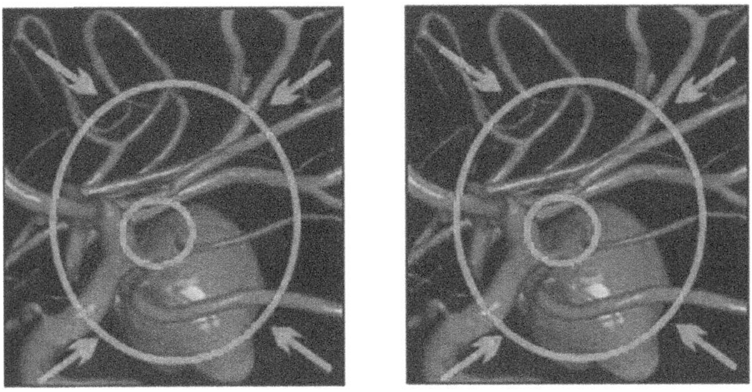

(D) (E)

FIGURE 13.7 (Continued)
Images (D and E) show enlarged images of breast cancer seen through LEVP along with REVP viewed through D3D. Note the several lines that point out the edges of breast mass. These display minor projections that stick out from the mass's surface. Since it points toward the user, the D3D scheme's depth sense is the only way to see the small circle inside the circle, indicating spiculation. For the best AR viewing experience, you need an HMD, which we havediscussed previously. It is possible to see both the real world and the virtual image simultaneously with this method. Note: The lines shown in the image were added to help visualize the complex arrangement of tissues. These lines will be automatically generated by a computer in the future. The 3D cursor, which was also computer-generated, had its size and placement over the tumour manually set by the user.

13.3 AR/VR'S FUTURE ROLE IN MEDICAL IMAGING

AR/VR could make medical images even better. Imaging is very important in chemotherapy for finding cancer, diagnosing it, and monitoring the treatment. During treatment, AR/VR technologies can be used to visualize multiple images of a tumour at different times to monitor changes in terms of size, shape, interaction with nearby structures, and edges. Tissue segmentation and extraction techniques isolate the tumour's outer boundary, making it possible to precisely compare how the tumour evolves over time. It is likely that the breast CT will get better at both spatial and contrast resolution, leading to larger image databases and a greater focus on image optimization, potentially enhanced via AR/VR visualization. AR/VR might also improve communication between the radiologist, oncologist, and surgeon.

Currently, the radiologist gives information about the location of the tumour, such as whether it is in the right or left breast, its size, and its position based on the clock-face method. However, augmented reality could improve this by providing more comprehensive information, such as the tumour's orientation, the 3D site of its spiculations, and its proximity to nearby anatomical structures. In particular, marking the edges of the tumour before surgery and using precise registration could help surgeons better understand the complex nature of the tumour and make it easier to remove the whole tumour during lumpectomies, while minimizing the risk of leaving behind residual cancerous tissue.

13.3.1 What Remain Some Possible Benefits of Using AR and VR?

Most importantly, there has not yet been a direct comparison between AR/VR and traditional volume rendering methods in medical imaging yet, so it's too early to say which is better. In theory, however, AR/VR could have advantages over traditional volume modeling methods, although these benefits have not yet been proven. For example, because AR/VR provides natural depth perception, it may reduce the need for complex computer processing required for volume rendering methods, such as generating artificial light sources and creating shadows from structures in the image. This could also reduce reading errors caused by image processing. The enhanced depth perception may help with imaging and identifying lesions, such as microcalcification patterns. Lastly, improved depth awareness might decrease the need for manual thresholding, making it easier to understand complex body structures faster and in more detail. Additionally, overlaying digital material on the image and enabling the doctor to use interactive processing tools might be more effective in an AR/VR setting. For example, tools such as computer-aided detection (CAD), customizable 3D cursor that can be any size and shape, false colour overlays to highlight various regions of the body, and arrows indicating the locations of micro-calcifications can help doctors communicate more effectively and improve interactions between patients and doctors. VR/AR technologies may make encourage wider use of the tools and methods listed earlier to enhance patient care as well as make it easier to manage large amounts of medical data.

The AR/VR earpiece enables enhanced human–controller interface capabilities. Some commercial headsets feature separate displays for each eye and can track head movements. For example, when the user turns their head to the right, the view shifts accordingly to the right; the same applies for upward and downward movements. Consequently, radiologists can swiftly comprehend a patient's anatomy and focus on specific areas of concern. An augmented reality device may be operated using controllers similar to those used in the gaming industry. The controller enables radiologists or end users to swiftly change viewing angles, zoom in or out, rotate, and manoeuvre the 3D pointer, among other functions. The AR/VR system offers significant potential advantages, reinforcing the earlier claim stated in this chapter. Primarily, it increases the likelihood of early tumour detection, since genuine 3D augmented reality allows for rotation, zooming, and navigation within the 3D volume, revealing tiny tumours that might have been obscured by traditional methods. True 3D augmented reality offers new possibilities for visualization, potentially enabling radiologists to get a clearer representation of abnormalities, such as the characteristic distribution of microcalcifications, thereby facilitating more accurate diagnoses. Collectively, these advancements could reduce misdiagnoses, improve patient care, alleviate patient worry, and lower healthcare costs. Future applications of AR/VR using D3D technologies might comprise complex imaging techniques, such as brain connectivity mapping with diffusion tensor imaging, combined positron emission tomographic (PET)-MRI scans, or advanced 3D facial recognition, analysis, and cosmetic enhancement.

13.3.2 The Problems of AR/VR vs Volume Rendering Persist

It is important to acknowledge that even though depth perception mitigates the issue of lapping constructions, it does not completely eradicate it. Second, as previously noted, a significant issue of virtual reality is motion sickness, which is associated with inadequate head tracking. Motion sickness may impair radiologists' care, perhaps leading to misclassification of key findings. Third, a significant problem is the integration of an HMD into the radiological reading room. An extensive study on virtual reality in surgery indicates that doctors will not embrace big head-mounted displays in the operating room.

13.4 CONCLUSION

This chapter examines CT and MRI image capture and traditional three-plane cross-sectional interpretation, and explores progressive 3D imagery methods such as surface rendering, volume rendering, D3D, VR, and AR. Comparative analysis of volume rendering and AR/VR has not yet been conducted; nonetheless, we examined the likely benefits and drawbacks of both methodologies. Examples were the identification of microcalcification patterns in breast cancer; quality evaluation of alterations in tumour morphology and borders; advancement of human–machine interfaces; and improved interaction between radiologists and physicians. Upcoming investigations in analytical imagery must contain comparative analysis of volume rendering, augmented reality, and virtual reality methodologies.

REFERENCES

1. Baetzner, Anke S., et al. "Preparing medical first responders for crises: a systematic literature review of disaster training programs and their effectiveness." *Scandinavian Journal of Trauma, Resuscitation and Emergency Medicine* 30.1 (2022): 76.
2. Pratticò, Filippo Gabriele, et al. "Exploring simulation-based virtual reality as a mock-up tool to support the design of first responders training." *Applied Sciences* 11.16 (2021): 7527.
3. Crane, Monique F., et al. "Developing resilience in first responders: strategies for enhancing psychoeducational service delivery." *Psychological Services* 19.S2 (2022): 17.
4. Way, David P., et al. "Learner evaluation of an immersive virtual reality mass casualty incident simulator for triage training." *BMC Digital Health* 2.1 (2024): 56.
5. Braun, Philipp, et al. "Virtual reality for immersive multi-user firefighter training scenarios." *Virtual Reality & Intelligent Hardware* 4.5 (2022): 406–417.
6. Du J., Q. Wang. Personalize wayfinding information for fire responders based on virtual reality training data. In *Proceedings of the 52nd Hawaii international conference on system sciences*, Grand Wailea, HI (2019).
7. Sai Sanjana K.B., K. Sai Mounika, T. Raja Santhosh Kumar, D. V. Srikanth. Thermal analysis of advanced IC engine cylinder. *International Journal of Automobile Engineering Research and Development (IJAuERD)* ISSN (P). 2016 Jun 30: 2277–4785.
8. Nofal, Abdullah R., et al. "Enhancing team performance through mock drills in disaster medicine and emergency medical services." *Journal of International Crisis and Risk Communication Research* 7.2 (2024): 265–275.
9. Rathore, P. S., S. Ahuja, S. R. Burri, A. Khunteta, A. Baliyan, & A. Kumar (2024). *Deep learning techniques for automation and industrial applications.* John Wiley & Sons, Inc.; Scrivener Publishing LLC.
10. Mukhopadhyay, Ayan, and Yevgeniy Vorobeychik. "Prioritized allocation of emergency responders based on a continuous-time incident prediction model." *International Conference on Autonomous Agents and MultiAgent Systems*, São Paulo, Brazil (2017).
11. Humphress, Rick. "Building an emergency response competency system: optimizing emergency personnel mobilization." *Journal of Homeland Security and Emergency Management* 4.3 (2007): 1–17.
12. Kumar, T., and R. Santhosh. "Design and Dynamic Analysis of Flywheel." *International Conference on Recent Innovations in Civil & Mechanical Engineering*, New Delhi, India, e-ISSN.

13. Matinrad, Niki, and Tobias Andersson Granberg. "Optimal pre-dispatch task assignment of volunteers in daily emergency response." *Socio-Economic Planning Sciences* 87 (2023): 101589.
14. Bongiovanni, Ivano, et al. "Implementation of best practices for emergency response and recovery at a large hospital: a fire emergency case study." *Safety Science* 96 (2017): 121–131.
15. Grochtdreis, T., N. de Jong, N. Harenberg, S. Görres, P. Schröder-Bäck. Nurses' roles, knowledge and experience in national disaster pre-paredness and emergency response: A literature review. *South Eastern European Journal of Public Health (SEEJPH)* 7 (2017).
16. Hawe, Glenn I., et al. "Agent-based simulation for large-scale emergency response: a survey of usage and implementation." *ACM Computing Surveys (CSUR)* 45.1 (2012): 1–51.
17. Paul, Nicholas R., Brian J. Lunday, and Sarah G. Nurre. "A multiobjective, maximal conditional covering location problem applied to the relocation of hierarchical emergency response facilities." *Omega* 66 (2017): 147–158.
18. Drezner, Jonathan A., et al. "Effectiveness of emergency response planning for sudden cardiac arrest in United States high schools with automated external defibrillators." *Circulation* 120.6 (2009): 518–525.
19. Zhou, Yang, et al. "Lagrangian relaxation-based approaches for cooperative location and assignment of emergency responders." *Alexandria Engineering Journal* 107 (2024): 225–234.
20. Frigstad, Lasse, et al. "Joint planning of drones and volunteers in emergency response to out-of-hospital cardiac arrest." *Computers & Industrial Engineering* 185 (2023): 109648.
21. Otal, H.T., E. Stern, M. A. Canbaz. Llm-assisted crisis management: Building advanced llm platforms for effective emergency response and public collaboration. In *2024 IEEE Conference on Artificial Intelligence (CAI)*, Marina Bay Sands, Singapore. 2024 Jun 25 (pp. 851–859). IEEE.
22. Harz, Christopher Robert, and Pamela A. Stern. *Serious games for first responders: improving design and usage with social learning theory (Volume A)*. Dissertation. Pepperdine University, 2008.
23. Coïsson, E., L Ferrari. Emergency response to damaged architectural heritage: Time, safety and conservation. In *International Conference on Structural Analysis of Historical Constructions*, Kyoto, Japan. 2023 Sep 4 (pp. 1320–1331). Cham: Springer Nature Switzerland.
24. Rainer, Karin, et al. "SimRad. NBC-simulation and information system for rescue units at CBRN disasters." *Intelligent Distributed Computing III: Proceedings of the 3rd International Symposium on Intelligent Distributed Computing–IDC 2009*, Ayia Napa, Cyprus, October 2009. Berlin, Heidelberg: Springer Berlin Heidelberg, 2009.
25. Segovia, R.O., A. Buelna, B. Sunderman. An examination of studies related to Brazilian jiu-jitsu in enhancing mental and physical health among veterans and first responders: A scoping review. *Sport Journal*. 2024 Aug 30. Available at https://thesportjournal.org/article/an-examination-of-studies-related-to-brazilian-jiu-jitsu-in-enhancing-mental-and-physical-health-among-veterans-and-first-responders-a-scoping-review/

Index

Pages in **bold** refer to tables and pages in *italics* refer to figures.

M

N

O

P

R

S

T

U

V

X